Treating Patellar Tendinitis with Strengthening Exercises

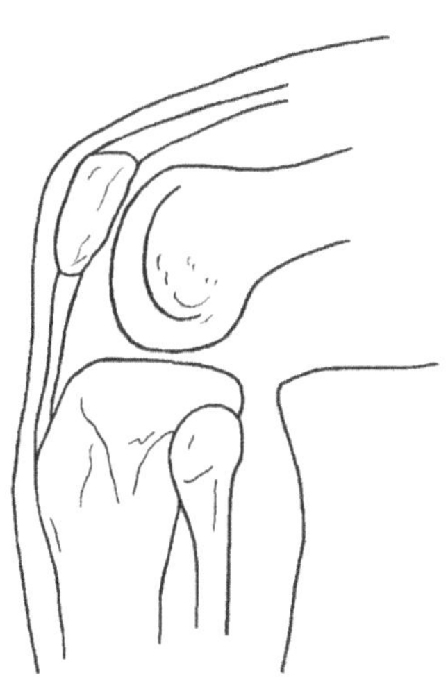

by

Jim Johnson, PT

Drawings by Eunice Johnson

I have given my best effort to ensure that this book is entirely based upon scientific evidence and not on intuition, single case reports, opinions of authorities, anecdotal evidence, or unsystematic clinical observations. Where I do state my opinion in this book, it is directly stated as such.

—Jim Johnson, P.T.

Table of Contents

①

BASICS

So your knee hurts and you've got patellar tendinitis. What exactly is that and how do you get rid of it?

Well, to begin with, if you're searching for information on patellar tendinitis in the medical literature, you won't find that much. Why? Because researchers changed the name awhile back to patellar *tendinopathy*. The problem was that the "itis" in tendinitis means that there's inflammation involved – which isn't really the case. But more on that later when we get into the nuts and bolts of the problem.

So in order to be more accurate, medicine switched the name from patellar tendinitis to *patellar tendinopathy* – and if you search the medical databases for information using that term, you'll find the bulk of the research there. Unfortunately, however, this "more correct" term hasn't really caught on with most people, so I'll still call it "patellar tendinitis" in this book just to avoid any confusion.

Anyway, a wise person once said, "If I had an hour to solve a problem, I'd spend fifty-five minutes thinking about the problem and five minutes thinking about solutions." The point here, of course, is that tough problems are much more easily solved when you *first* understand them. So with that in mind, let's start with the very basics of how your knee is put together. Now instead of just listing all its parts, and then giving you some boring medical definitions, I think it's much more interesting to go over the knee's structures by taking a look at pictures of it from the *inside* out. Up first is the basic framework of your knee, *the bones…*

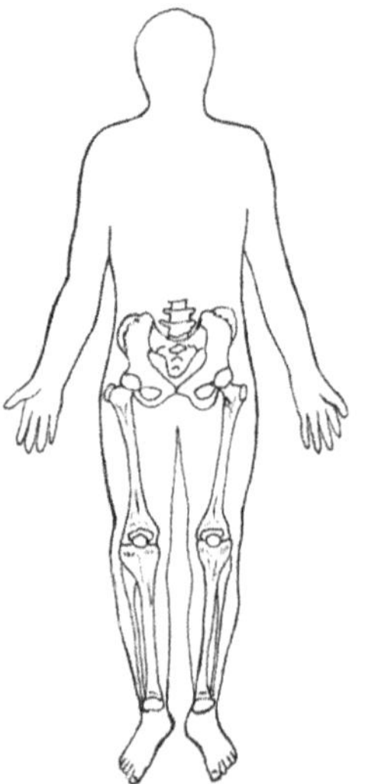

**Figure 1. The bones of the upper and lower leg
that come together to form your knees.**

A look at Figure 1 quickly tells us that the knee is made up of more than just one bone. The following gives us a closer look, and reveals to us that the knee is actually made up of four distinct bones; the *femur* (upper leg bone), the *tibia* (the lower leg bone), the fibula (smaller lower leg bone) and the *patella* (your kneecap).

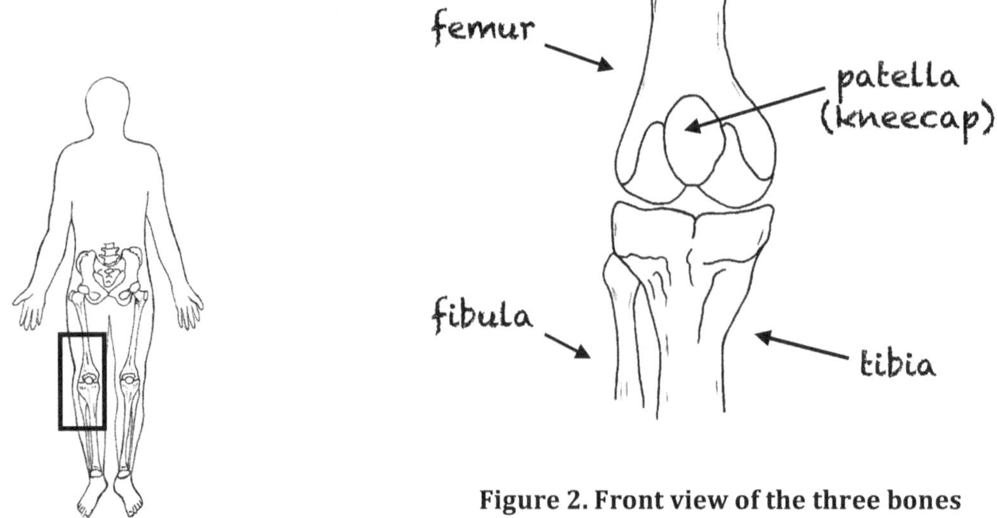

**Figure 2. Front view of the three bones
that make up the *right* knee joint.**

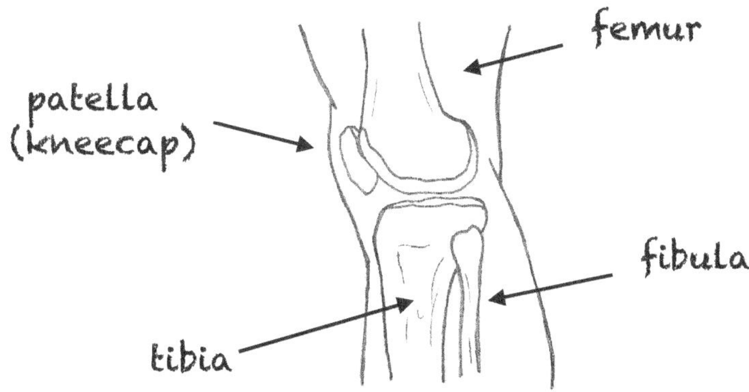

**Figure 3. Side view of the four bones
that make up the *left* knee joint.**

The Articular Cartilage

Now that you have an idea of what bones make up your knee, it's important to note that where they do come together and meet, their ends are coated with a substance called *articular cartilage.* Being super slick and very smooth, it's a big job of the articular cartilage to decrease friction between the bones and help them move smoothly upon one another. Here's a side view showing where the articular cartilage coats the ends of your knee bones…

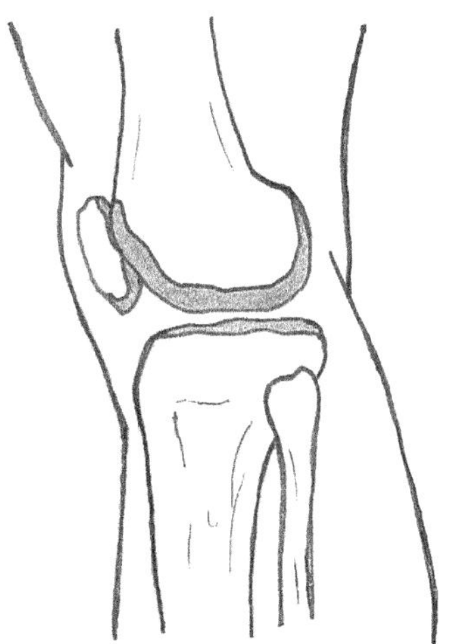

**Figure 4. Shaded areas show where the knee bones
are coated with smooth articular cartilage.**

Here are a few more pictures at different angles. This one is good because it shows the cartilage that is located on the *back* of your kneecap. Yep, you've got cartilage there too!

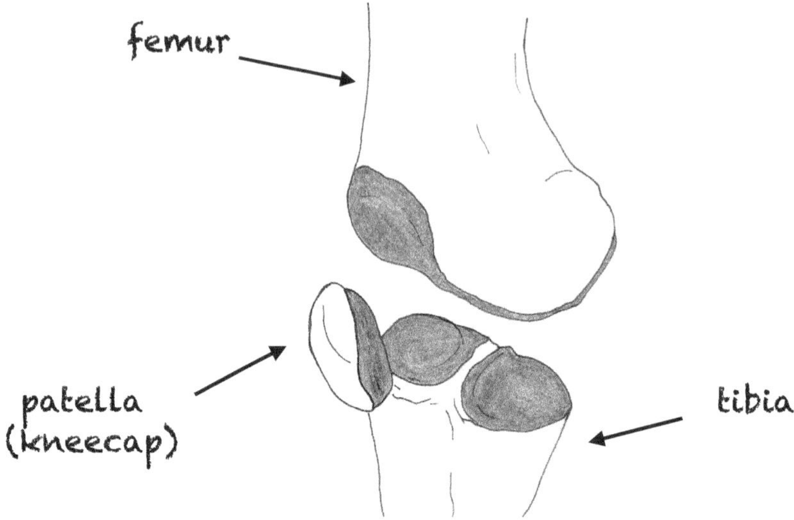

Figure 5. Shaded areas show where the articular cartilage is.

And this one shows the areas of cartilage with the kneecap removed and the knee in a *bent* position.

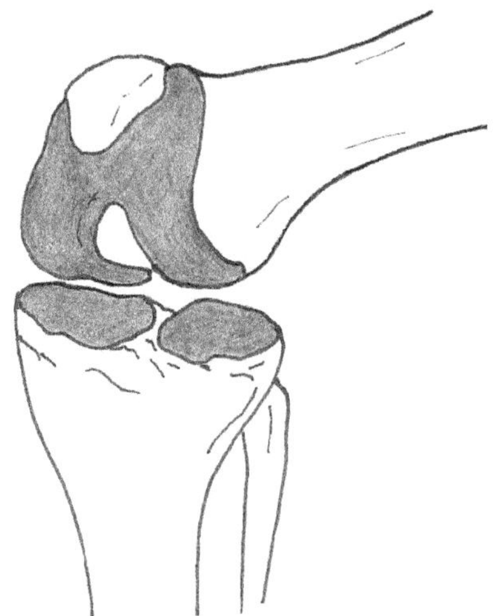

Figure 6. Shaded areas show where the articular cartilage is.

Know that normal articular cartilage is a white, smooth, firm substance that is made up of cells called *chondrocytes*. However unlike other tissues in your body, like the skin or muscles, articular cartilage has *no* blood supply going to it. In other words, there are no small blood vessels going directly to it to provide life-sustaining nutrients. So just how do these tiny little chondrocytes get their nutrition?

To answer that question, we have to take a microscopic look at how the articular cartilage is made up. If you take a piece of articular cartilage from your knee joint, and look at it from the *side* under a powerful microscope, you'd see that it actually has several different layers to it. Check out this picture and you'll see what I mean…

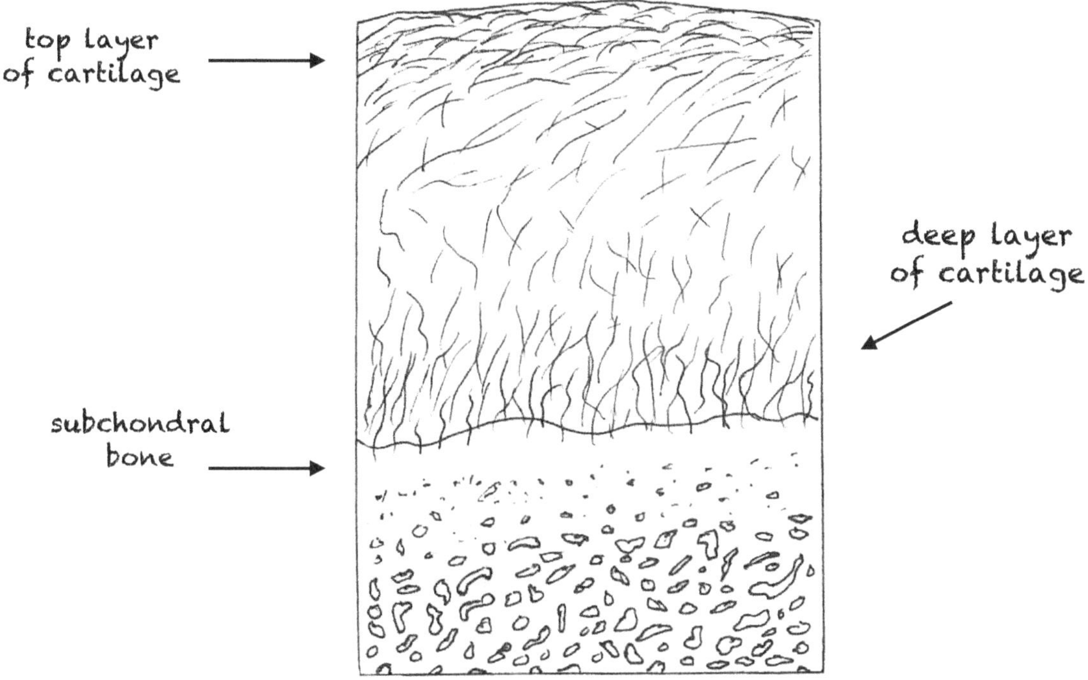

Figure 7. A side view of the different layers of the articular cartilage in the knee. Note how the knee cartilage eventually blends with the underlying bone.

As you can easily see, there are several different layers to the articular cartilage. Scientists believe that the top layer gets its nutrition from a liquid floating around in the knee joint known as *synovial fluid* (more on that stuff in a few pages).

And the deeper layer of cartilage? It's most likely that it gets its nutrition from the *subchondral bone* it's right next to. In case you're confused, the subchondral bone is just a fancy name for the bone that sits *right under* the layers of cartilage.

The Meniscus

Now even though the ends of the tibia and femur are coated with this super-slick articular cartilage stuff that helps them move smoothly upon each another, you can see looking back at Figure 6, that the ends of the two bones are shaped *very* differently from each other – not exactly what you'd call "a perfect fit."

So, in order to help this situation, there are two little structures *in between* the two bones called the *medial meniscus*, and *the lateral meniscus*. Pronounced mun-iss-cuss , here's what they look like sitting in your knee…

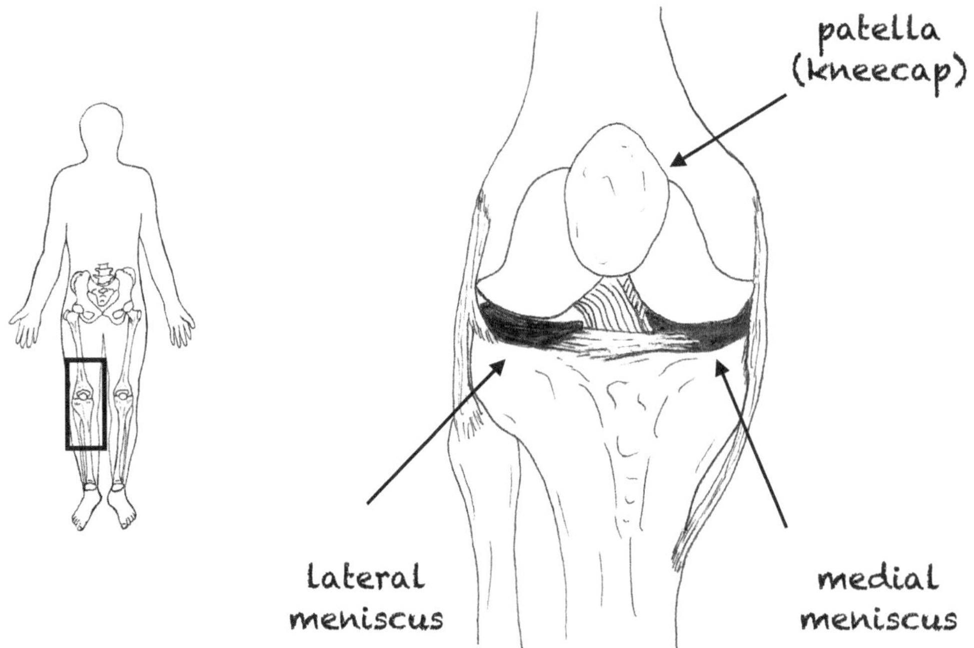

Figure 8. Front view of the medial and lateral meniscus of the right knee.

Since the upper bone of the knee, the femur, has two *round* parts that sit directly on the *flatter* tibia bone, you can see how the medial and lateral meniscus really help to improve the fit between the two bones.

Now that you've seen what the medial and lateral meniscus look like from the front, let's lift up the femur a bit to get a better look at things…

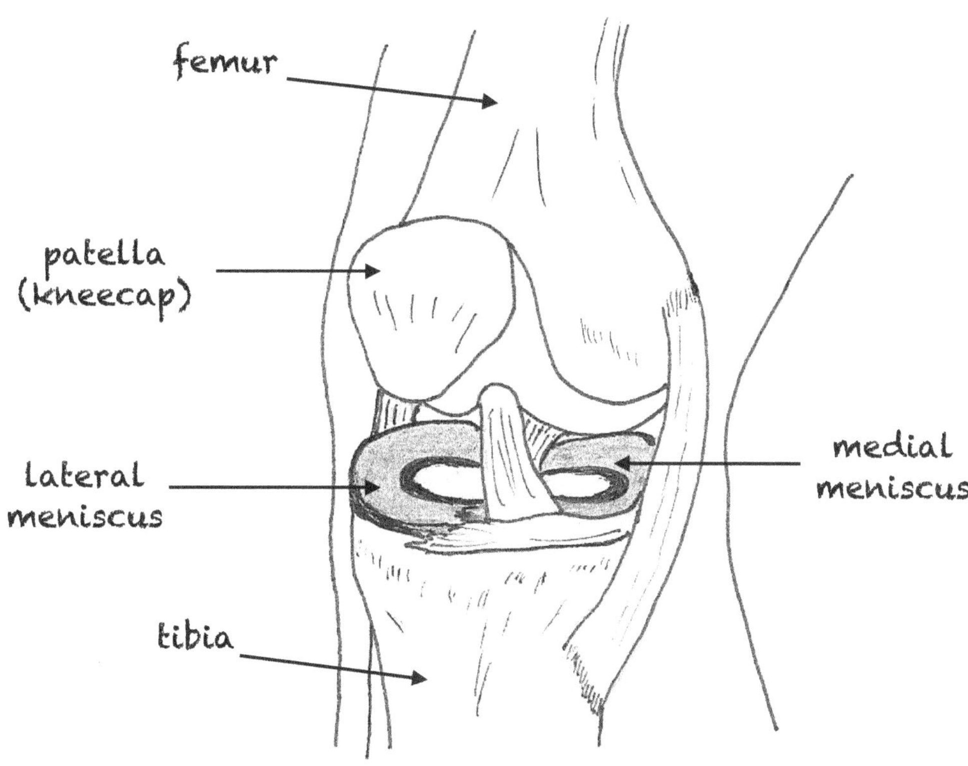

**Figure 9. How the medial and lateral
meniscus sit in the right knee joint.**

Like the articular cartilage that coats the end of the bones, the medial and lateral meniscus are also made of cartilage - however it's a different kind called *fibrocartilage*.

Besides helping the femur and tibia fit together a little better, the medial and lateral meniscus also help out with shock absorption and work hard to transmit forces across the knee more efficiently. This last picture reveals how different the medial and lateral meniscus really are in shape…

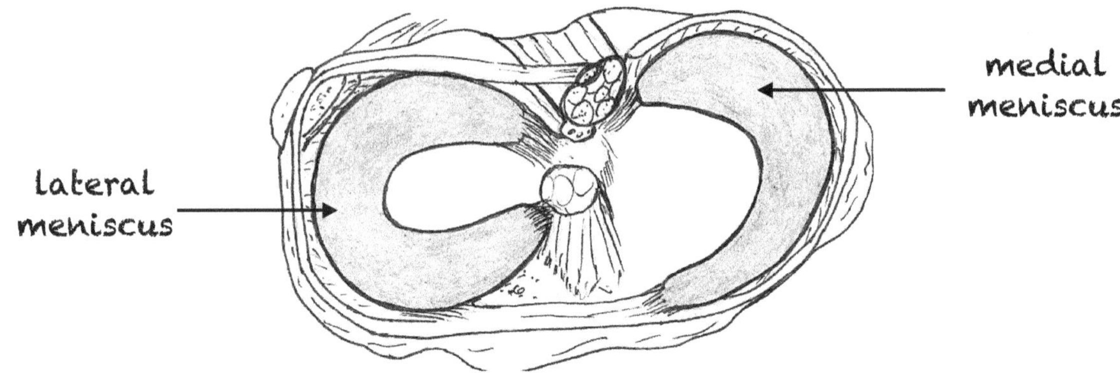

**Figure 10. Overhead view of the
medial and lateral meniscus.**

The Ligaments

Okay. Up to this point we've got two bones covered with smooth articular cartilage on their ends, that are neatly fitted together with two pieces of fibrocartilage in between them. So the next question is, what keeps them together? Well, it's a specialized connective tissue known as a *ligament.*

While there are many different ligaments in and around the knee, some big, some small, we're going to take a look at the major ones. There are four of them, and they are:

- the anterior cruciate ligament
- the posterior cruciate ligament
- the medial collateral ligament
- the lateral collateral ligament

Since it's the job of the ligaments to hold the bones together, it's logical that they'd have to run from one bone to another. Let's see exactly where they are in the knee…

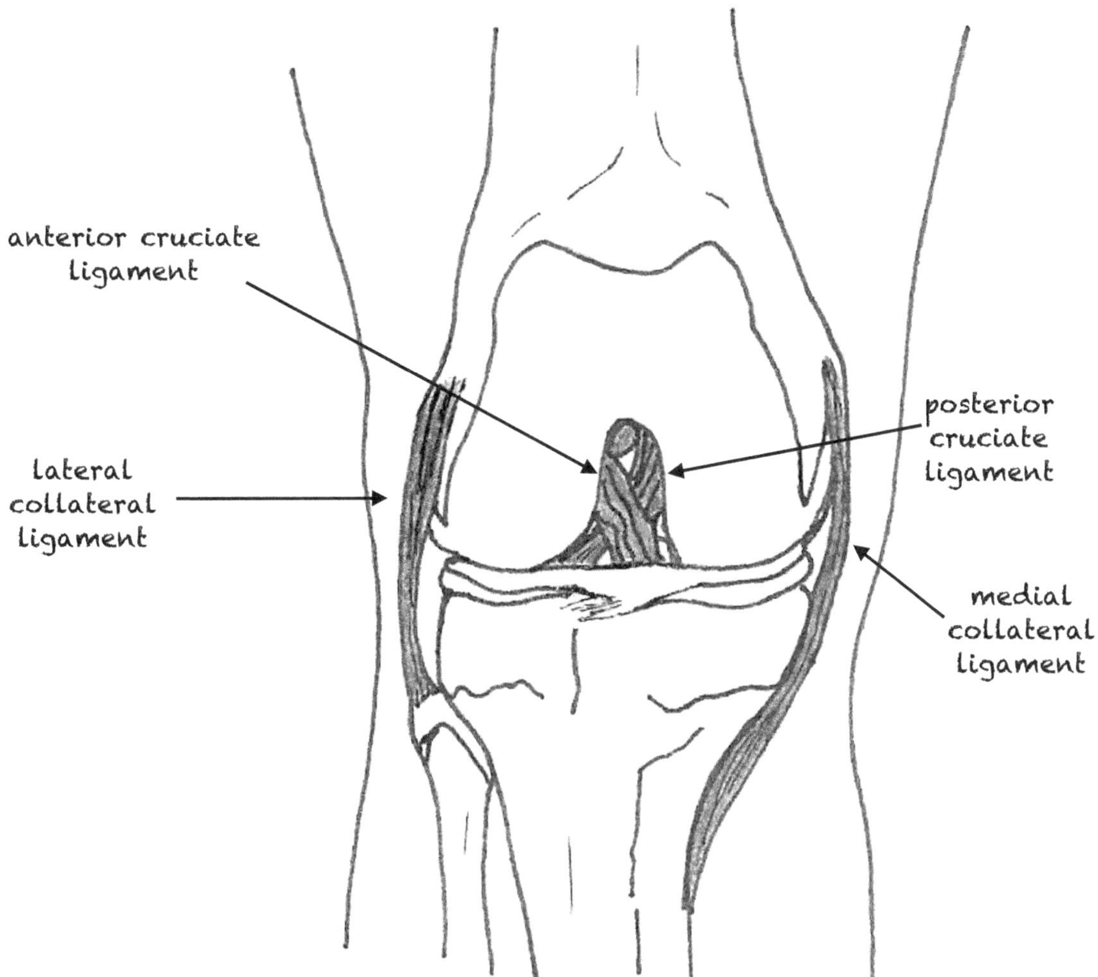

Figure 11. Front view of the four major ligaments of the right knee that help hold the bones in place.

Did you notice that the two ligaments in the middle cross each other and make an "x"? That's why they were named the *cruciate* ligaments, because "cruciate" comes from the Latin word "crux" – which means cross. By the way, if you've ever heard of an athlete tearing their "ACL", it was the Anterior Cruciate Ligament that they tore. Ouch!

While these four ligaments work hard all day to help hold your knee bones in place, don't think that they just sit there stiff as a board. If that were the case, you wouldn't be able to move your knee around very much!

So just how do these ligaments work? Well, a ligament will allow a certain amount of motion to take place in the knee, but, if a bone starts going *too far* in one direction, growing tension in the ligament stops it. By working this way, the ligaments can both *permit* a certain amount of knee motion, as well as *limit* it. Take a look at these examples and you'll see how the ligaments react as you move your knee around…

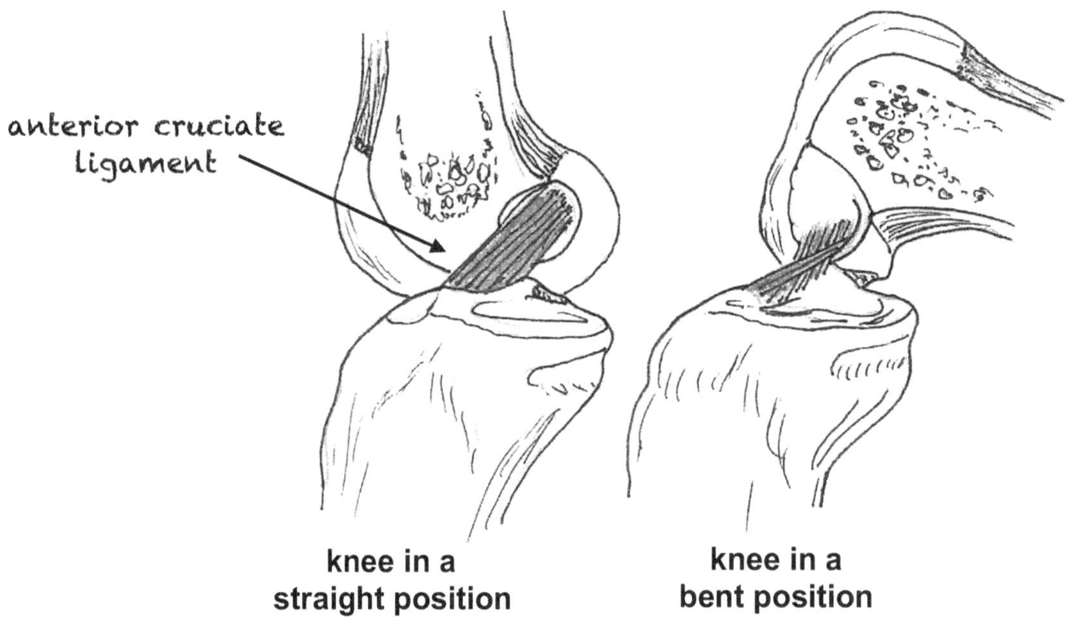

Figure 12. A side view showing how the
anterior cruciate ligament reacts when
you bend and straighten your knee.

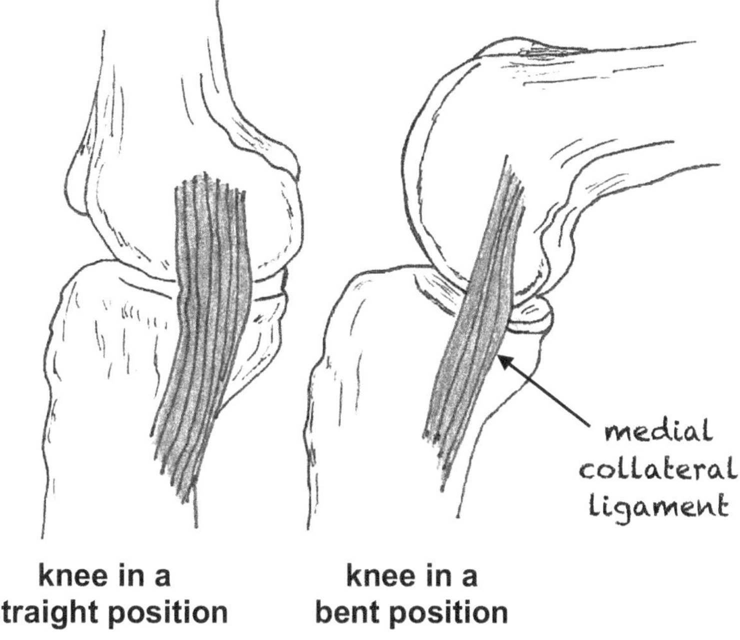

Figure 13. A side view showing how the
medial collateral ligament reacts when
you bend and straighten your knee.

The Synovial Membrane

I doubt a lot of readers have heard of this knee structure. The *synovial membrane* is like a "sleeve" that fits neatly around your knee joint and envelopes it. This is what it looks like :

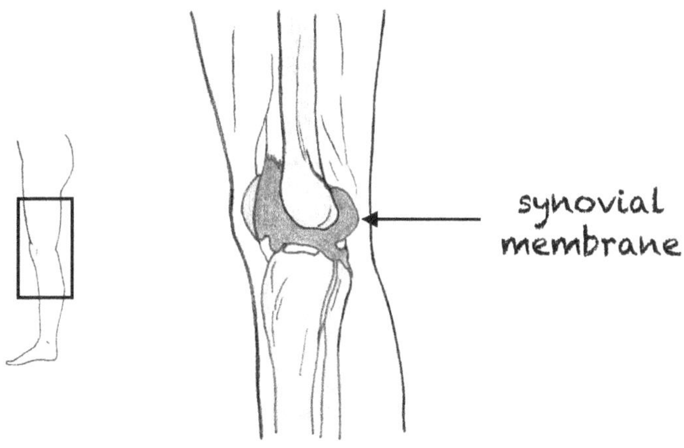

Figure 14. The synovial membrane

Interesting structure, isn't it? Think of the synovial membrane kind of like a plastic wrap that clings closely to the entire knee joint. Here are a few more pictures to give you a better lool

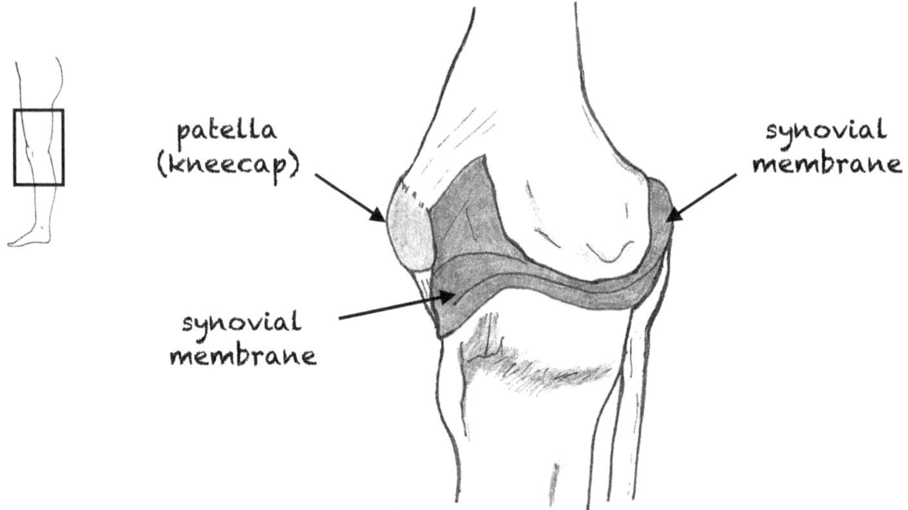

**Figure 15. A side view of
the synovial membrane**

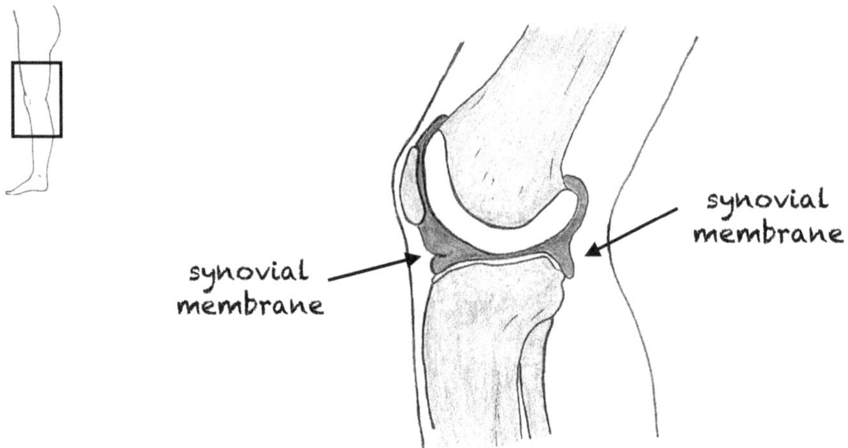

**Figure 16. A cutout side view of the synovial
membrane. Note how the synovium wraps itself
around the two bones and "seals in" the knee joint.**

So what does the synovial membrane do? Well, it lines the joint and makes that substance we talked about on page 6 called *synovial fluid*. Synovial fluid is a must-have to your knee, because it floats around and provides nutrients to the cartilage in your knee. Additionally, it also helps lubricate your knee joint.

The Bursae

Have you ever heard of bursitis? A lot of people have. It's common in the shoulder, and you get it when you have a problem with a small structure called a *bursae* (pronounced burr-sah). So what's a bursae?

Well, bursae in general are flat, sac-like structures that are located *all* throughout your body. If you've ever seen a deflated whoopie cushion, well, that's about what they look like. It's the main job of these bursae to reduce friction and make things slide a whole lot easier, particularly in areas where structures have a tendency to rub together a lot – like where a tendon passes right over a bone.

Now normally these little guys contain a small amount of fluid, however if they get really irritated for any number of reason, well, they can really swell up and cause you a lot of pain – and then you've got bursitis. You've got a bunch of bursae around your knee joint, and here's a picture of some of the major ones…

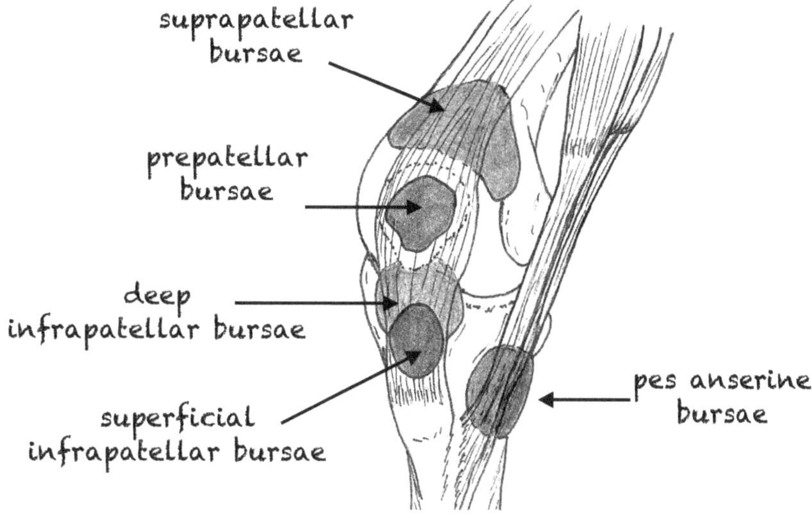

Figure 17. Some of the major bursae around the right knee.

The Muscles

We're finally to one of the last and outermost structures of your knee, the muscles – which make your knee move. While there are quite a few of them in and around the knee, I just want you to be familiar with two major groups in particular – the *quadriceps* and the *hamstrings*. As the following pictures show, the quadriceps muscles take up most of the *front* of your thigh, while the hamstrings make up most of the *back*. Here's a look at where they are…

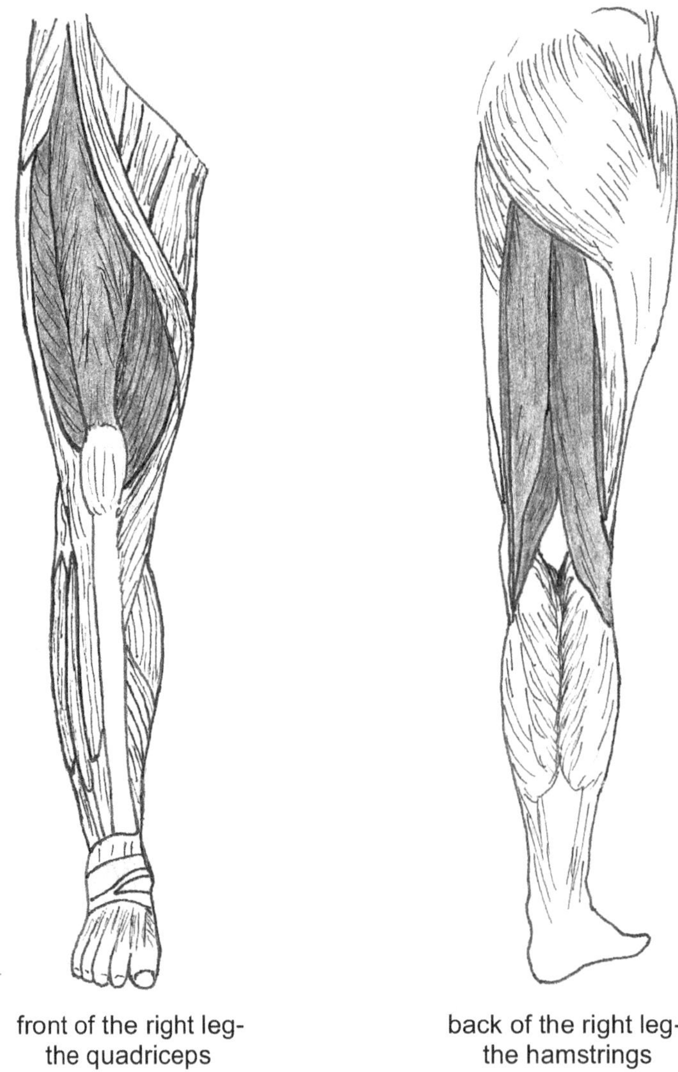

Figure 18. Shaded areas showing the quadriceps and hamstring muscle groups.

Now as most people already know, it's the job of these muscles to move your legs. This is accomplished by the muscles contracting and getting shorter – which in turn pulls on the bones and creates movement so you can walk, run, etc. However, muscles don't attach themselves to the bones directly. Instead, you have a specific type of tissue called *tendon*, which connect the muscles to the bones. And the tendon we're most interested in here, of course, is your *patellar tendon*. Here's where it's at…

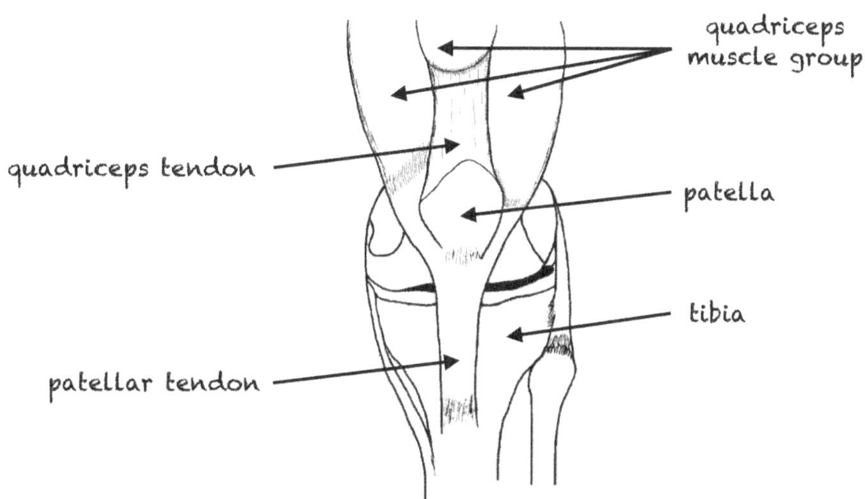

Figure 19. The location of the patellar tendon in the left knee.

So if you follow the picture from the top down, you can see the quadriceps muscle group connecting right to the quadriceps tendon. The quadriceps tendon, in turn, attaches to the patella (your knee cap) – and running from the patella to the tibia is the patellar tendon. Here's a look from the side…

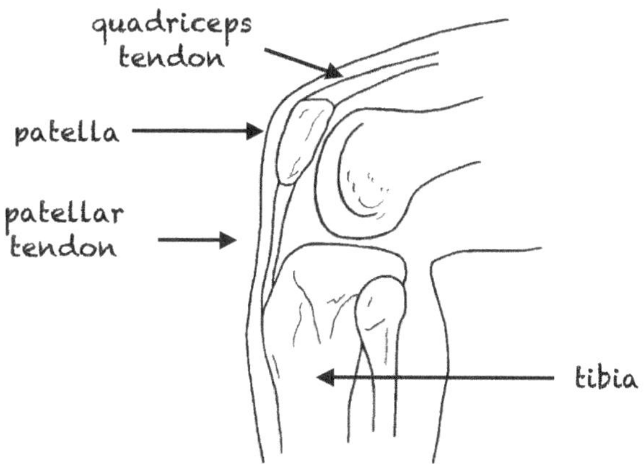

Figure 20. Side view of the patellar tendon in the left knee.

Finding your patellar tendon is easy because it sits *right* under the skin. If you look down at your straightened knee, the circle shows you where you can press down and put your finger *directly* on it…

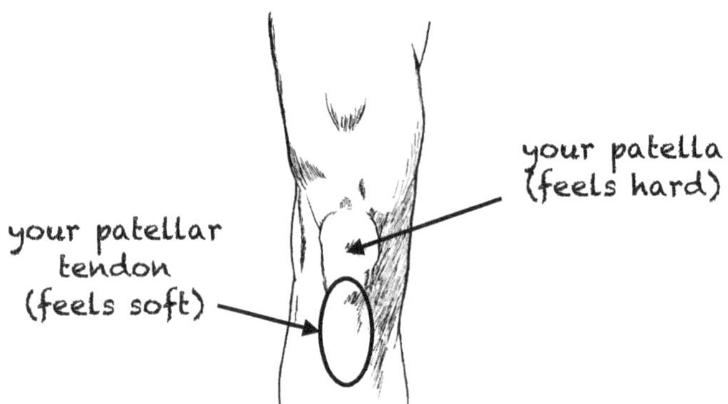

Figure 21. Finding the patellar tendon in your right knee.

In the above picture, you can see a *vague* outline of your patellar tendon – but if we looked right *under* the skin, here's what you'd find…

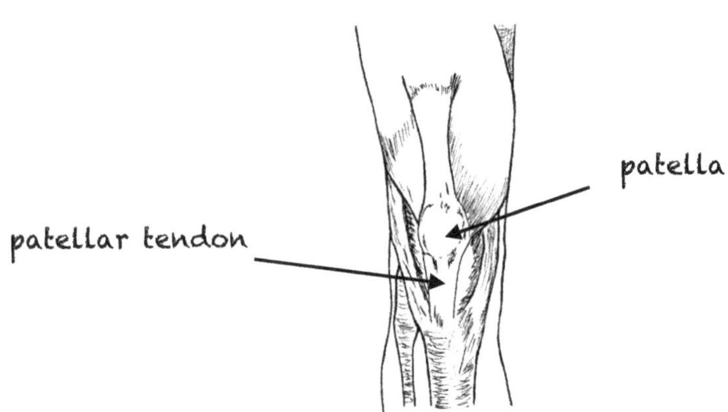

Figure 22. Directly beneath the skin of the right knee.

As we mentioned earlier, tendons connect muscles to bones, and as you can guess from all these pictures, it's the job of your patellar tendon to help connect the *quadriceps muscle* to your *tibia bone*. This is why you can confirm that you're actually feeling your patellar tendon by simply lifting your foot in the air, or kicking your foot out while your finger is on it – your patellar tendon will tighten up as the quadriceps muscle pulls on it.

What does the quadriceps muscle do?

Because the patellar tendon is being pulled on *all the time* by *the quadriceps muscle*, and its force is being transmitted through it, it's important to know what the quadriceps muscle (or "quads") actually does.

Probably the best way to explain its function is to sit in a chair and kick out your leg. This action is one of the main jobs of the quadriceps muscle, that is, it helps you straighten out your leg. Now try this. Stand up from a sitting position, and as you do so, put one hand on the front of your thigh. You should be able to feel the muscles under your hand (the quadriceps) tighten and firm up as you begin to rise. This is yet another important function of this muscle. With your foot fixed on the floor as you stand up, the quadriceps muscle works to pull you into a standing position. Along with these activities, your quads are also largely responsible for your ability to walk, run, jump, and climb stairs.

②

THE CAUSE

As I mentioned earlier, the term "patellar tendinitis" was changed some time ago to "patellar tendinopathy" – the reason being that researchers failed to find any inflammation in patients with patellar tendinitis. So since this inflammation myth is still quite popular, let me explain the facts in a little more detail…

What the Microscope Tells Us About Patellar Tendinitis

Approaching this matter scientifically, as we do everything in this book, to say that something is "inflammed" means that we should be able to find some hard evidence of inflammation. Without getting too caught up in details, inflammation can be broken down into two general patterns, *acute* and *chronic*. Here is the difference between the two:

- *acute inflammation* is an immediate and early response to tissue injury. It comes on quick, but lasts for minutes, hours, or a few days. Neutrophils are the major kind of cells that are involved in acute inflammation.

- *chronic inflammation* is inflammation of a prolonged duration, such as weeks or months. Some of the major types of cells that are involved in chronic inflammation include macrophages, lymphocytes, and plasma cells.

Now it's *not* important to know all about the different types of cells, although you may be interested to know that a lot of them are simply different types of white blood cells. What is important, however, is to know that these are exactly the kinds of cells we should be able to find in people with patellar tendinitis *if* the tendon or muscle is indeed "inflammed"– since these are the cells directly involved in the body's inflammatory process.

Throughout time, however, the vast majority of studies have most certainly *failed* to find any. For instance, here's a few of them from the published literature where researchers have taken a piece of the patellar tendon in people with "patellar tendinitis" and analyzed it…

study	*# of patients*	*duration of symptoms*	*reported histological findings*
Fu 2002	**11**	**more than 6 months**	**"inflammatory cells could not be identified"**
Alfredson 2001	**5**	**12-36 months**	**"there were no inflammatory cell infiltrates"**
Popp 1997	**9**	**more than 2 years**	**"most notably absent from all of the specimens were any cysts or acute inflammatory cells"**
Khan 1996	**24**	**mean 35 months**	**"inflammatory cells were not seen in any specimen"**
Yu 1995	**9**	**3 years on average**	**"no acute inflammatory cells were present in any of the specimens"**

Well, as you can see from the above table, it doesn't look like researchers have reported finding any of the cells that are directly involved in the inflammatory process. Therefore, without some cellular proof of an inflammatory response, one has *no basis* to accurately say that there is indeed "inflammation" when one has patellar tendinitis - the evidence just isn't there! Unfortunately, even though these (and many more) studies have been out for literally years, the information hasn't seemed to have gotten around like it should. So beware of using anti-inflammatory creams or any other treatments whose purpose is to get rid of inflamation in your knee that simply isn't there!

> ***Critical point***: Inflammation does *not* appear to be a major feature of patellar tendinitis, especially in patients that have been suffering with this condition for many months.

On the other hand, what researches *have consistently found* when taking a piece of tendon at surgery, and looking at it later under a microscope, are signs of **failed tendon healing**. Here are three of the most common findings...

- *disrupted and disorganized collagen fibers.* Collagen is a main ingredient that makes up your connective tissues – and it's having a hard time coming together properly in the tendon!

- *fibroblastic proliferation.* Fibroblast cells work like a "construction crew" to make connective tissue. We see a lot of these little guys, some abnormal, floating around in the tendons of patellar tendinitis sufferers – so they're obviously looking for work!

- *vascular proliferation.* Lots of blood vessels, many of which are abnormal and immature, are found in the area – a sign that tendon healing is trying to take place!

But enough written descriptions. Let's take a look at a few drawings to get a better "picture" of what's going on...

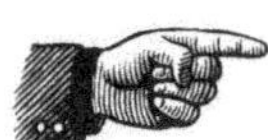

Here's what a normal patellar tendon looks like under a microscope…

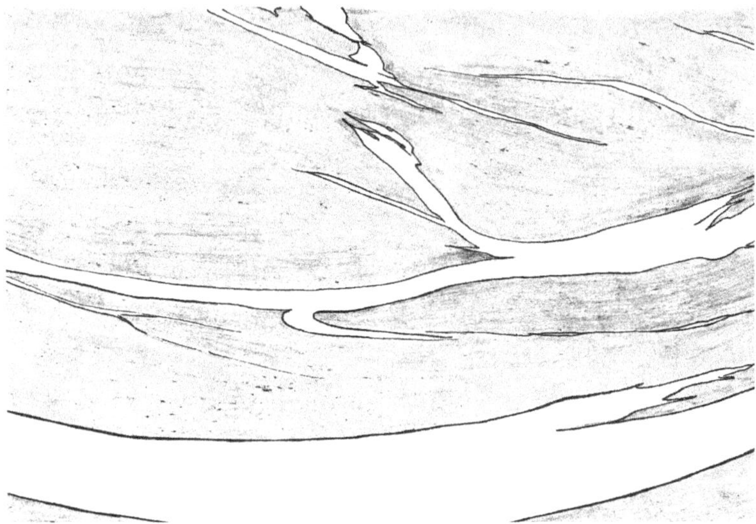

Notice how straight and *organized* the tendon fibers are. That's the way things are *suppose* to be. Now check out this drawing…

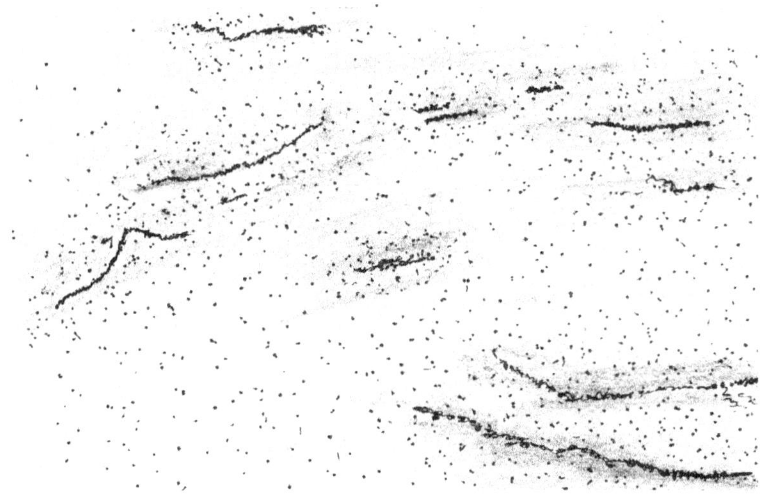

Wow! And that's what your patellar tendon looks like when you have patellar tendinitis. Looks a little different from the first one, doesn't it? What a mess! As you can tell, there's *a lot* of disorganization going on there. Your body is trying to repair itself - but can't quite get its act together. But how did the tendon become so abnormal?

How Patellar Tendons Get Messed Up

The answer to the question, "How did the tendon become so abnormal?" can be answered in one word: *overuse*. The story goes something like this.

First, know that as you use your legs throughout the day, you're contracting the muscles, which are in turn pulling hard on your tendons (remember that tendons help connect the muscles to the bones). And, just like most things in your body, the tendons and muscles need time (at some point) to rest and repair themselves from this normal daily wear and tear.

Therefore, if you work your tendons and muscles, and give them *enough* time to recover each day, they're going to stay in good shape. We could then say that your muscles and tendons are "keeping up" with your activities. And all is well.

Now let's say you have a day where you've worked your tendons and muscles *more* than normal, or you're just using them in a way they're simply not used to. For example, maybe you did a lot more running that day, or maybe you just tried a new sport after work like volleyball. Well, of course this is going to cause *more* wear and tear than the muscles and tendons are normally used to, right?

Well, here's where problems can start. **If** you give your leg muscles and tendons time to rest and recover (meaning that they have time to make the necessary repairs from this increased stress) *before* using them a lot again, your tendons will be able to "keep up", stay in good working order, and will continue looking like this…

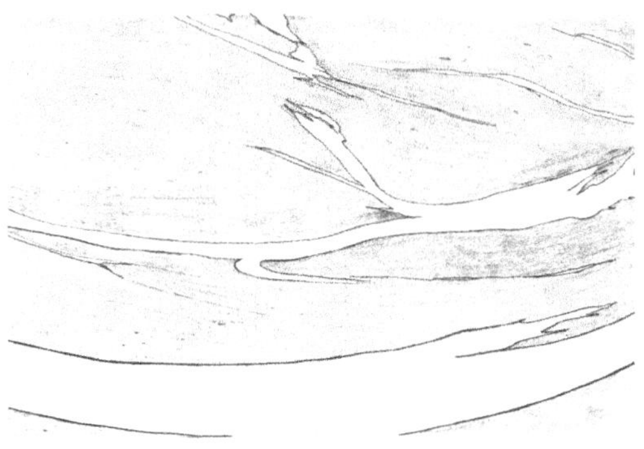

On the other hand, let's say you *continue* to repeatedly work your muscles and tendons harder than usual and they don't get enough time off to recover and make repairs. What will happen to them then? Well, *over time* your tendons will be unable to "keep up" with the activities you ask them to do, start to become internally disorganized, and will eventually end up looking like this...

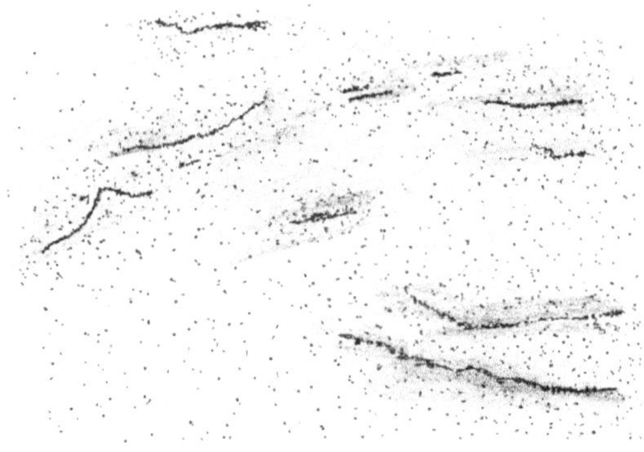

The moral of the story? The main problem in patellar tendinitis is one of **failed tendon healing**. And the tendon has failed to heal because it was repeatedly put through stressful activities – and then not given enough repair time.

③

THE CURE

So if the cause of patellar tendinitis is an overstressed tendon, the first obvious thing to do would be to stop overstressing it - by eliminating (or lowering) the harmful stresses that are being placed on it. Doing this sets up the right environment for the tendon to begin its healing process. This means that if running is the activity that overstressed your patellar tendon, you need to cut back, or altogether stop running. Likewise, if jumping is the offending activity, decreasing or stopping it will definitely facilitate healing.

However it isn't always possible to pinpoint or eliminate the offending activity(s), which brings us to perhaps the best strategy of all – *improving the quality of your patellar tendon tissue.*

The Healing Changes That Need To Take Place

Improve the quality of the patellar tendon tissue. Hmm. What exactly does that mean? Well, recall from the last chapter…

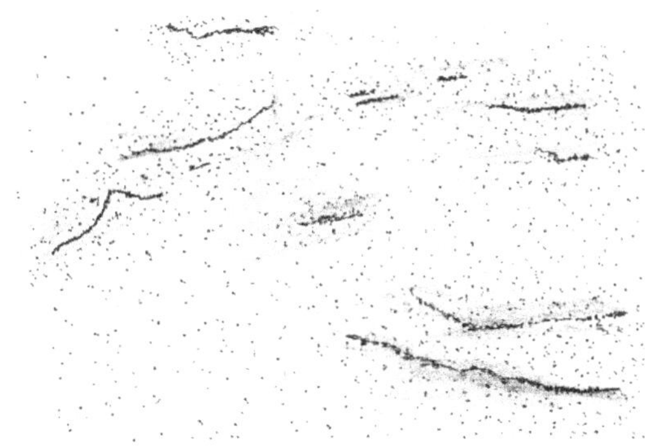

This is what your patellar tendon looks like *now*.

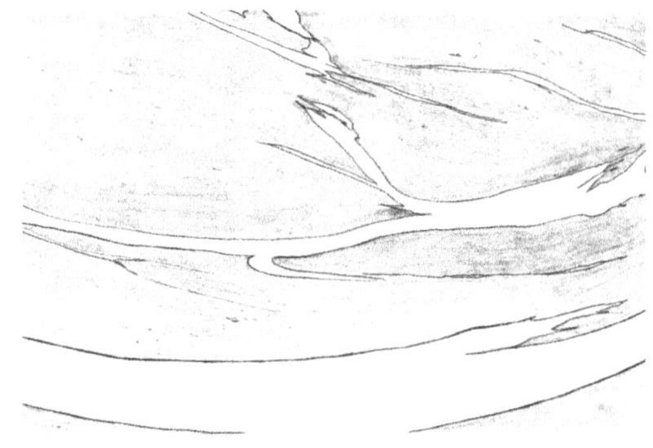

This is what your patellar tendon *needs* to look like.

The goal is to get from the picture on the left to the picture on the right. But how? Well, by *reversing* the disorganized changes that have taken place. So what we need here is a treatment that can…

✓ **encourage a new blood vessel supply**

✓ **promote the formation of healing tissue cells (such as fibroblasts) and healing materials (such as collagen)**

✓ **make the newly formed tissue line up properly**

If we can somehow "jump start" things, and make these changes begin to happen, well, it'll be just a matter of time before your patellar tendinitis heals up. But is there one single treatment that can pull all of this off? Actually there is. Physical therapists have been using many different types of *strengthening exercises* for years to successfully treat patellar tendinitis – let me give you a short summary of each…

Number 1: Eccentric Decline Squats

The first type of strengthening exercise that became popular to successfully treat patellar tendinitis is called the *eccentric decline squat*. Of course you already know what "decline" and "squat" means, but what's *eccentric*?

Well, it describes the *type* of muscle contraction used in this particular strengthening exercise. While most people are aware that your muscles contract to make your arms and legs move around, it's not common knowledge that there are actually *several* kinds of muscle contractions – each one working a little differently.

How many are there? Three: *concentric, eccentric,* and *isometric* muscle contractions. Since a picture is worth a thousand words, let me explain by using a couple of them…

Concentric Muscle Contractions

As you lift something, the muscle bunches
up and gets *shorter* as it contracts.

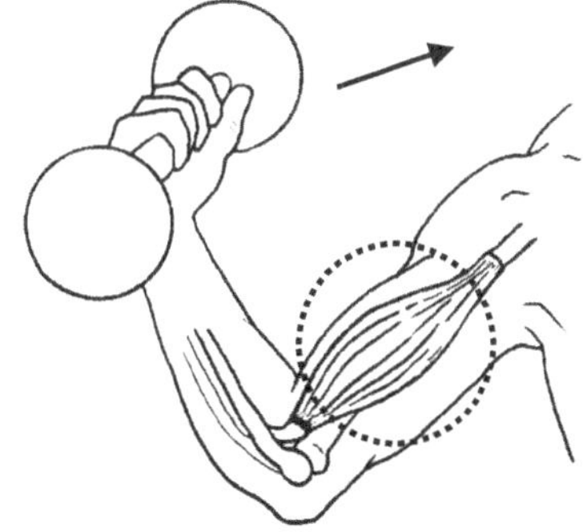

Eccentric Muscle Contractions

As you lower something, the muscle gets
longer and *lengthens* as it contracts.

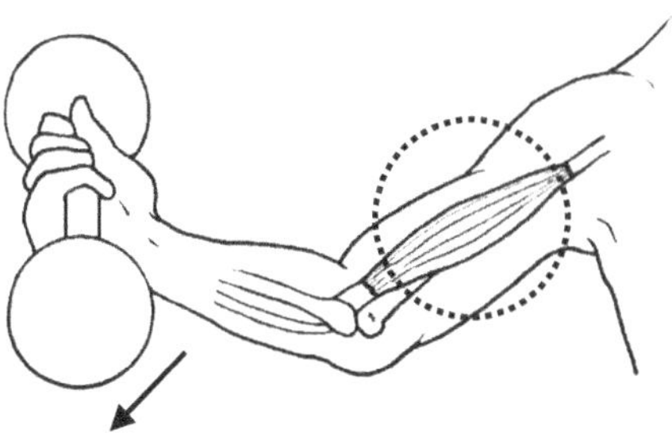

As you can see, when a muscle is contracting and getting shorter, we call it a *concentric* contraction. And, when the muscle is contracting and getting longer, we call it an *eccentric* contraction.

The third type of muscles contraction is called an *isometric* muscle contraction. The word *isometric* comes from the two Greek words *isos*, meaning "equal" or "like," and *metron*, meaning measure. An isometric exercise, then, is one in which the length of the muscle stays the same as it is contracting. A good example of this is when you use your hand and arm to push hard against a brick wall. Your arm is still and unable to move because you can't push the wall over, yet, there is a definite building up of tension in your muscle.

Isometric Muscle Contractions

As the dumbbell is being held still,
the muscle *stays the same length* as it contracts.

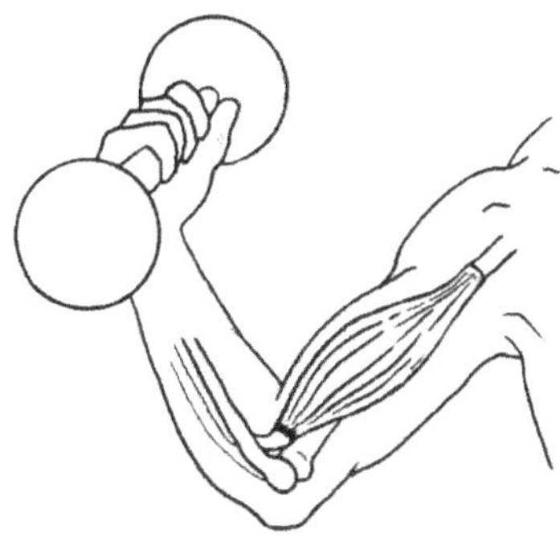

Okay, so now that you know what an eccentric contraction is, and how is differs from the other two types of muscle contractions - back to the eccentric decline squat. As you might have figured out by now, this exercise involves standing on a declined surface, which in this case is a slanted board, and squatting down. Here's how it's done…

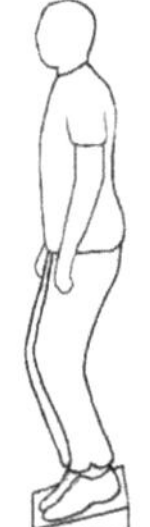

Stand on both legs on a slant board.

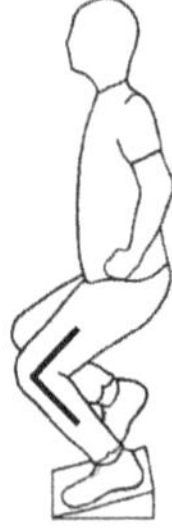

Using ONLY your knee with patellar tendinitis, squat down slowly, bending the knee to 90° (should take you about 2-3 seconds).

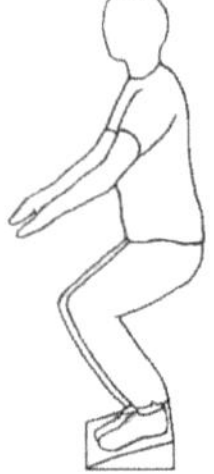

When your knee with patellar tendinitis has bent to 90°, stand on both legs.

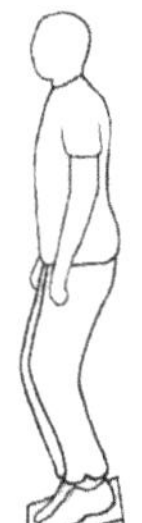

Now come back up to the standing position, USING YOUR GOOD LEG ONLY - as much as possible. Repeat. It is okay to feel pain while doing the exercise - but the pain should not be disabling.

The point of the eccentric decline squat is to squat down on one leg, the one with patellar tendinitis - which is an eccentric contraction of the leg muscles. Then, you raise back up to the standing position using just the other leg as much as possible. So why can't you use *both* legs to push back up to the standing position?

Well, because there is research showing that exercising a leg with patellar tendinitis using *just eccentric* muscle contractions (the squatting down part), produces much better results than using *just concentric* muscle contractions (the coming up from a squatting position part). For instance…

- researchers studied 15 patients that had patellar tendinitis (Jonsson 2005)

- 8 patients were randomized to do just the lowering part of the squat (eccentric group)

- 7 patients were randomized to do just the raising up part of the squat (concentric group)

- both groups used a 25° slant board

- 12-week follow-up showed that those in the eccentric group had a significant decrease in pain, while those in the concentric group showed *no* significant decrease in pain

- long-term follow-up (mean 33 months) revealed that patients in the eccentric group were still satisfied and sports active, while *all* patients in the concentric group had been treated surgically or with injections

A few points about the above study. First of all, it's a *randomized controlled trial*. In medicine, this research method produces the highest form of proof showing whether or not a treatment really works. In this book, I only cite results from randomized controlled trials, the best of the best evidence - to back up treatments for patellar tendinitis.

Another interesting thing to note is that the study used a 25° slant board – which is actually the most common angle used in the vast majority of studies on patellar tendinitis and eccentric decline squats. But why 25°? Why not 30° or 40°? Well, it turns out 25 isn't exactly a "magic" number...

- in this study, researchers tested 5 subjects doing the eccentric decline squat at varying decline angles (Zwerver 2007)

- decline board angles of 0°, 5°, 10°, 15°, 20°, 25°, and 30° were tested out

- force plates were used, as well as special equipment to measure joint angles in the leg

- results showed that angles greater than or equal to 15° *all* resulted in a significant increase in maximum patellar tendon force – *therefore, decline angles between 15° and 30° can be used to increase patellar tendon force* (which is the goal of the eccentric decline squat)

- furthermore, decline angles of greater than or equal to 35° were not practical as subjects slid downwards and couldn't stand upright

So now you're in the know. However despite the fact that other decline angles will stress the patellar tendon just as well, the eccentric decline squat done at a 25° decline continues to be the most tested. In fact, it's even gone head to head with *surgery*...

- in this randomized controlled trial, 40 knees with patellar tendinitis were divided up into two groups (Bahr 2006)

- 20 knees were randomized to have surgery

- 20 knees were randomized to perform the eccentric decline squat using a 25° slant board

- at 12-month follow-up, both groups improved – there was no measurable difference between the two groups

- The conclusion? Researchers found no advantage demonstrated for surgical treatment compared to the eccentric decline squat

---

Chalk another one up for the eccentric decline squat! If you want to give this exercise a try, I've already shown you *how* to do it – so here are some guidelines that are commonly used in randomized controlled trials that have shown the eccentric decline squat to be effective...

- ✓ do two sessions of the eccentric decline squat a day
- ✓ each session, do the exercise on p.28, squatting down 15 times in a in a row on the leg with patellar tendinitis. Rest a minute or so, then repeat 2 more times. You'll be doing a total of 3 sets of 15 reps per session – work up to it if you need to.
- ✓ when you can do 3 sets of 15 reps with minimal to no pain, increase the weight by 10 pounds at a time using a backpack. Repeat this process as necessary.
- ✓ continue the eccentric decline squat for 12 weeks

But what do you do if you have patellar tendinitis in *both* legs? Well, since we want to avoid doing the raising (concentric) part of the squat with either leg, the only other option is to assist this raising part somehow. Perhaps the easiest way is to use two chairs, like these pictures below show…

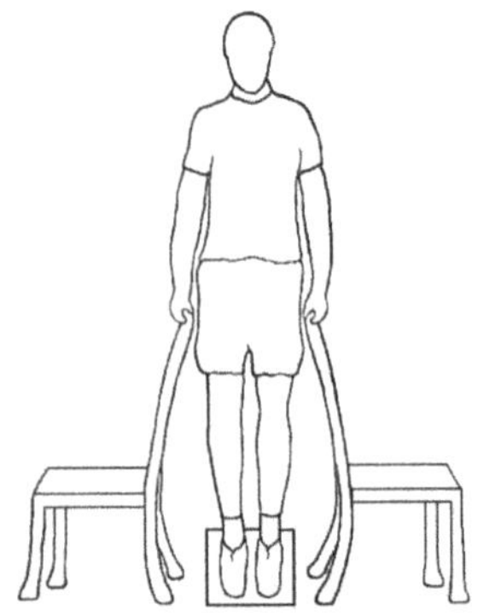

Okay, you start in this position, and then squat down slowly, bending both knees to 90°.

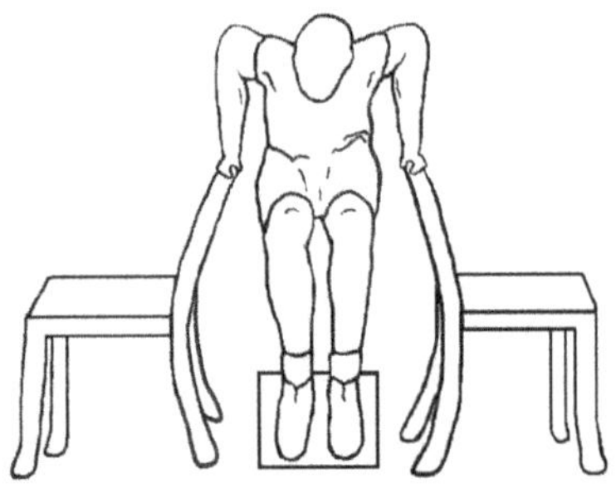

When both knees are bent to 90°, *use your arms as much as possible to raise yourself back up to the starting position.*

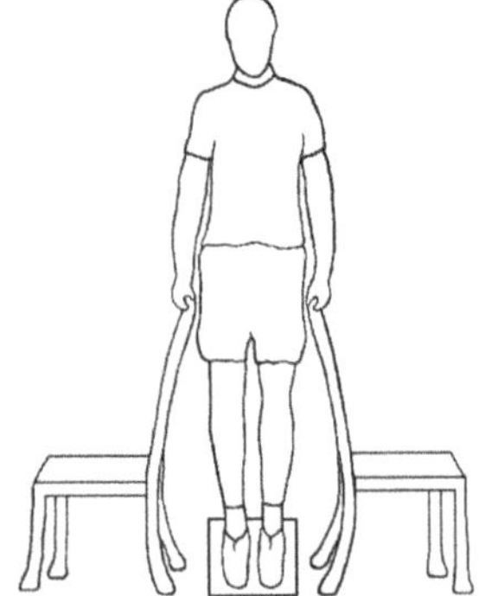

Repeat. Use the same guidelines as the single leg eccentric decline squat (3 sets of 15 reps twice a day, etc.)

Number 2: Heavy Slow Resistance Exercises

The eccentric decline squat, with its proven effectiveness in randomized controlled trials, quickly gained popularity. It was a matter of time, however, until researchers began testing out other exercises…

- 39 patients with patellar tendinitis were randomized to one of three groups (Kongsgaard 2009)

- the first group got steroid injections to the patellar tendon

- the second group did eccentric decline squats using a 25° slant board

- the last group did *heavy slow resistance exercises*

- patients were assessed at 0-weeks, 12-weeks, and 6-months

- researchers found that the group that got cortisone injections had good short-term, but poor long-term clinical results

- both the eccentric decline squat group, and the heavy slow resistance training group improved

- however, those in the heavy slow resistance training group were more satisfied with their treatment, and patellar biopsies showed that they had increased collagen turnover

This study shows us that cortisone injections do help, but the results are not long lasting at all – a common result in other overuse injuries as well, such as tennis elbow. But while both exercise groups significantly improved, and stayed better over the long run (unlike those that got the cortisone shots) – those in the *heavy slow resistance* group were more satisfied and had more normal patellar tendons in the end. So what exactly is this "heavy slow resistance training"? Well, it involves *three* exercises…

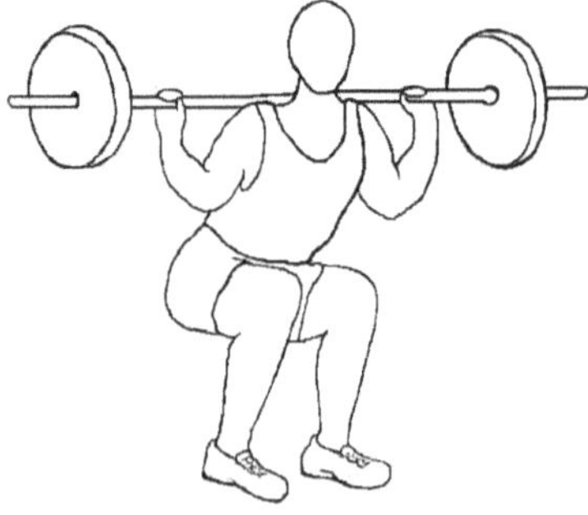

The Squat

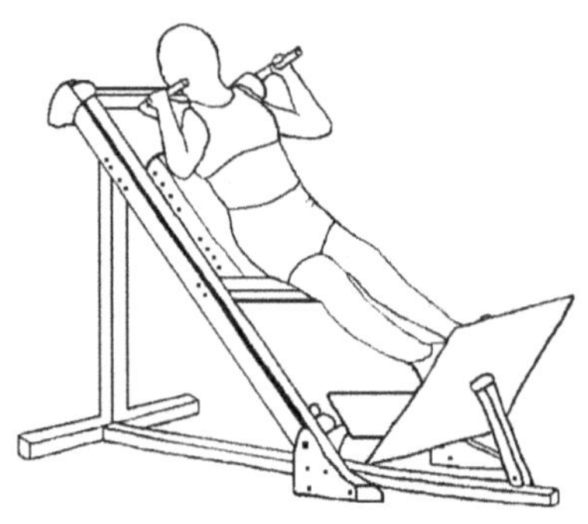

The Hack Squat

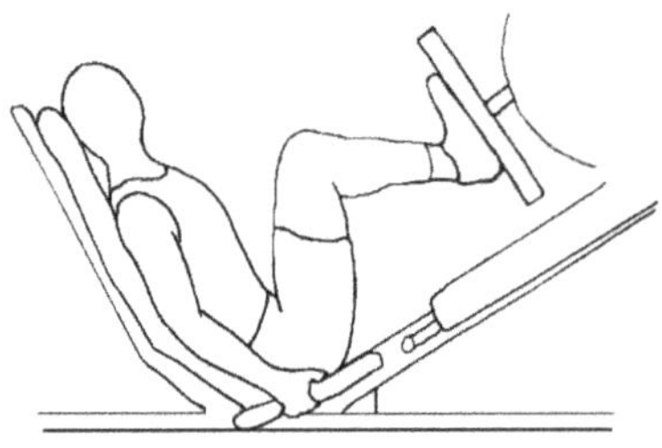

The 45° Leg Press

The following pages will show you how to do each one...

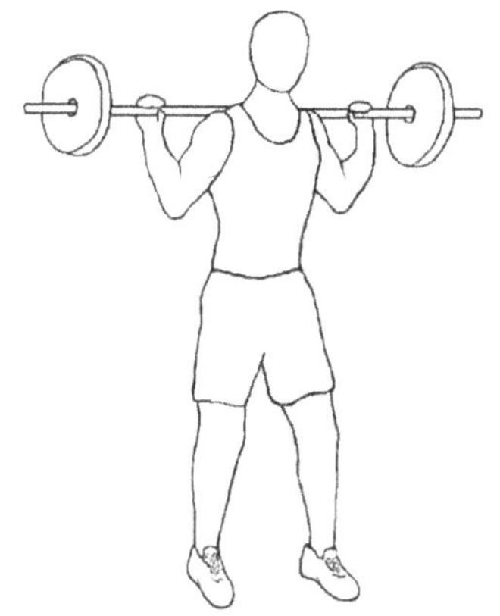

- Begin with a barbell across your upper back, gripping it with both hands as in the picture. Getting to this position is accomplished by using a squat rack – consult a professional in your gym if you don't know how to do this.

- Keep your back straight.

- Feet should be around shoulder width apart.

- Keep your foot position natural as this has no noticeable effect on muscle activity of the knee muscles.

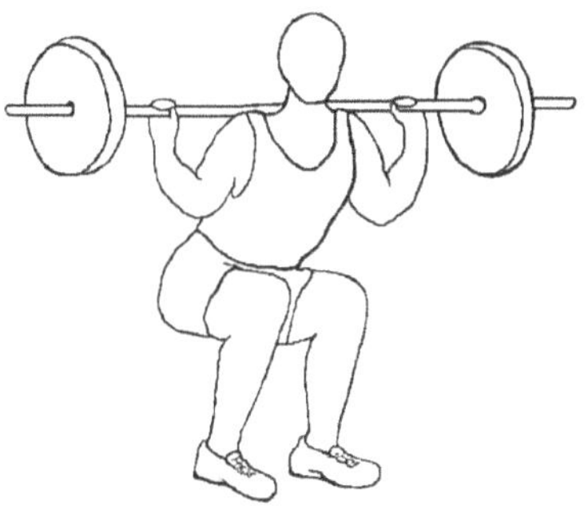

- Next squat down, bending your knees to a 90-degree angle, as if you were "sitting down in a chair."

- Keep your back straight.

- Make sure your knees do not pass beyond your toes as you squat down – this decreases stress on the knee.

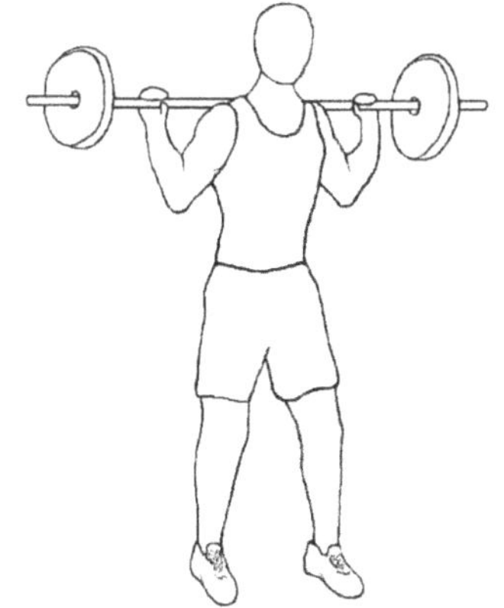

- Now come back up to the starting position – do not lock your knees, but rather keep them slightly bent.

- Repeat

- Speed: Take 3 seconds to bend knees, and 3 seconds to raise back up.

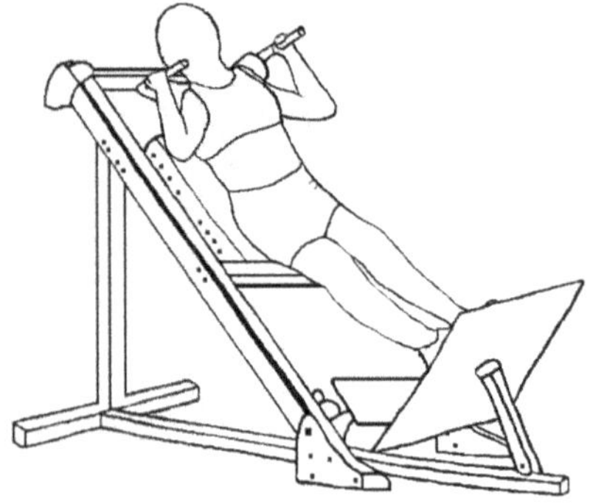

- Get into the starting position as shown, knees should be slightly bent.
- Position yourself with the feet on the uppermost portion of the platform – be sure your feet are forward of the body when positioned.
- Keep your back straight.
- Feet should be around shoulder width apart.
- Keep your foot position natural.

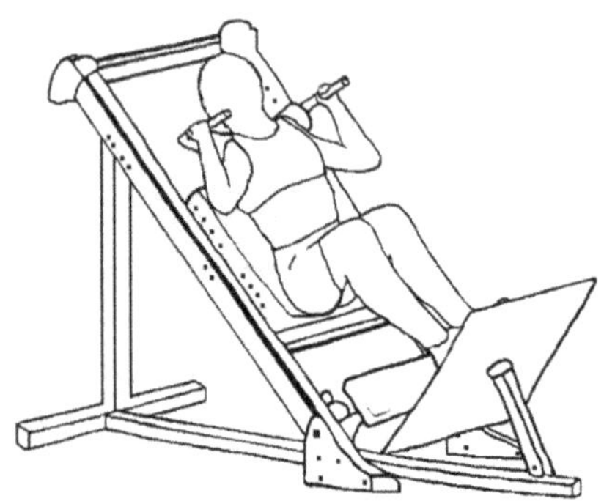

- Release the safety lock apparatus.
- Next, bend your knees to a 90-degree angle.
- Keep your back straight.
- Make sure your knees do not pass beyond your toes as you squat down. Standing towards the uppermost portion of the platform makes this possible.

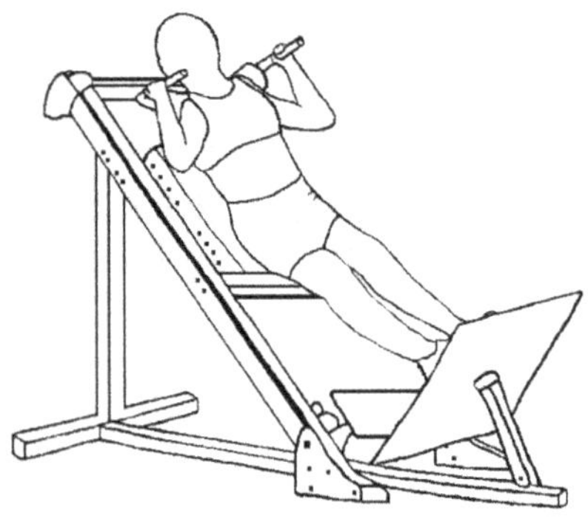

- Now come back up to the starting position – do not lock your knees, but rather keep them slightly bent.
- Repeat
- After finishing a set, engage the safety lock apparatus.
- It is recommended to first go up and down a few times with no weight so you can find the correct foot position on the platform - so that the knees don't go over your toes when squatting
- Speed: Take 3 seconds to bend knees, and 3 seconds to raise back up.

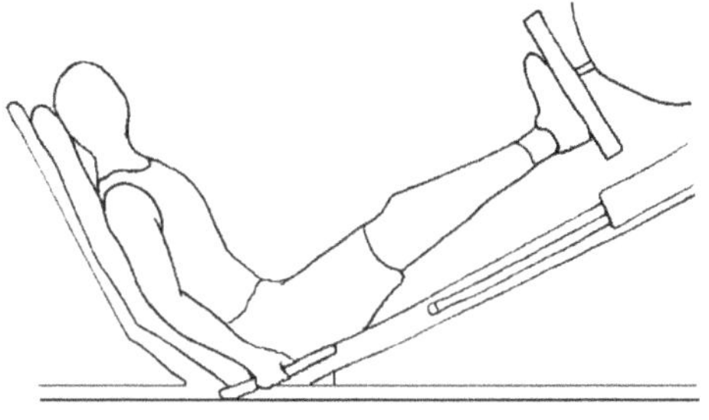

- Get into the starting position as shown, knees should be slightly bent.
- Position yourself with the feet placed around the middle of the platform.
- Keep your back straight.
- Feet should be around shoulder width apart.
- Keep your foot position natural.

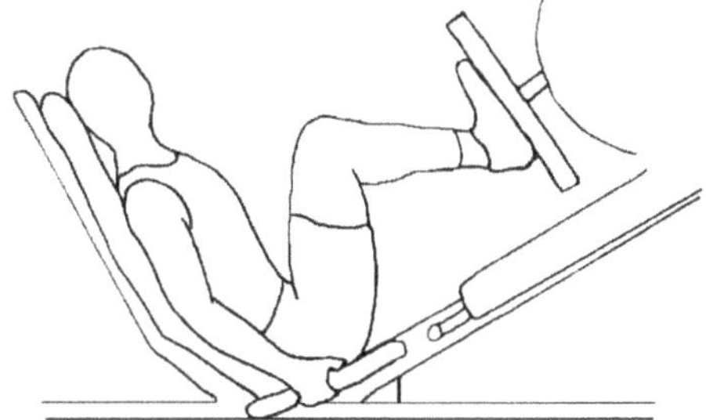

- Release the safety lock apparatus.
- Next, bend your knees to a 90-degree angle.
- Keep your back straight.
- Make sure your knees do not pass beyond your toes as the knees bend. Placing your feet around the middle of the platform makes this possible.

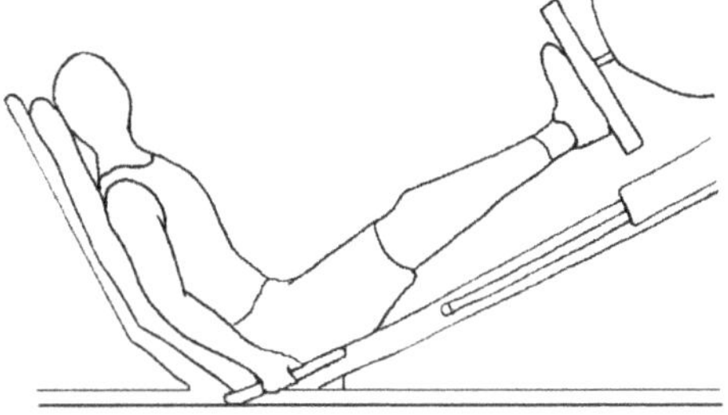

- Now push back up to the starting position – do not lock your knees, but rather keep them slightly bent.
- Repeat
- After finishing a set, engage the safety lock apparatus.
- It is recommended to first go up and down a few times with no weight so you can find the correct foot position on the platform - so that the knees don't go over your toes.
- Speed: Take 3 seconds to bend knees, and 3 seconds to push back up.

So there you have it - the exact exercises used in the study with people suffering from patellar tendinitis - which resulted in a better outcome and a more normalized patellar tendon compared to those doing eccentric decline squats.

Now if you've never done any of them before, it is suggested that you first consult with knowledgeable staff at your gym in order to get familiar with them. The exercise guidelines used in this 12-week program are as follows…

- all three exercises are done 3 times a week (i.e. M–W–F or T–TH–Sa)
- exercises are done with *both* legs
- do four sets of each exercise – with a 2–3 minute rest in between sets
- pain *during* the exercises are acceptable, but pain and discomfort should not increase after cessation of training
- sporting activities are allowed during the training period IF they can be performed with only light discomfort

And what about repetitions? Well, here's where it gets a little tricky, as these researchers used *repetition maximums*. And what's a repetition maximum?

Well, as an example, a one-repetition maximum is the most amount of weight you can lift one time, *and only one time* – lifting it twice is not possible. A two-repetition maximum, is the amount of weight you can lift just twice, and so on. Therefore, if you can lift 100 pounds only once, your one repetition maximum (1 RM) would be 100 pounds.

Now that you know that, here's the repetition numbers used week-by-week…

> - Week One: 4 sets of each exercise, each set using a 15 RM, 3x week
> - Weeks 2-3:   4 sets of each exercise, each set using a 12 RM, 3x week
> - Weeks 4-5:   4 sets of each exercise, each set using a 10 RM, 3x week
> - Weeks 6-8:   4 sets of each exercise, each set using an 8 RM 3x week
> - Weeks 9-12: 4 sets of each exercise, each set using a 6 RM, 3x week

As you can imagine, it takes a little trial and error to figure out a particular repetition maximum for a given week for each of the three exercises. For example, let's say you want to try this 12-week heavy slow resistance program and its Week One – so you have to find your 15 RM maximum for the squat, hack squat, and 45° leg press.

Starting with the squat, you first take a guess at what you think your 15 RM might be, and then test it out after doing a few warm-up reps with a really light amount of weight. So if you try to squat 100 pounds, and can do only 15 reps – you're set – you do four sets of 15 reps using 100 pounds during Week One, three days that week.

On the other hand, if you couldn't do 15 reps, rest a few minutes and try another set after either adding or subtracting weight - depending on if you did more or less than 15 times. Repeat this process until you eventually find the amount of weight you can do just 15 times. And of course, you'd also have to use this method to find your 15 RM for the hack squat, and 45° leg press as well for that week.

So looking at the outline above, when Week One is over, your new repetition maximum for Weeks 2 and 3 has now changed to a 12 RM. Therefore, you would simply use the same trial and error process just described to find your 12 RM for the squat, hack squat, and 45° leg press.

Continue using this trial and error process every week that you have a new RM during the 12-week program. Note that this also means that you'll be lifiting heavier and heavier weights throughout this 12-week program - because the weight you use for a 6 RM *is much heavier* than the weight you'd use for a 15 RM. That's because you can lift a lighter weight more times than a heavier weight!

As I mentioned, it *does* take a little trial and error, and some people may find it too tedious a process, or simply too much trouble to mess with. However, it *is* an option – and it has yielded some good results in a randomized controlled trial, making it well-worth mentioning. Now if heavy slow resistance training doesn't appeal to you, don't worry, there are more options…

Number 3 and 4: Isometric and Isotonic Leg Extension

The latest and greatest exercises being researched to treat patellar tendinitis involve leg extension. To extend your leg is to straighten it out – and this motion can be used several ways to treat patellar tendinitis. The first method involves getting in a sitting position, extending your leg partially, and then holding it there (an isometric exercise). The second way, also done in sitting, involves extending your leg until it is all the way straight – and then lowering it all the way down (an isotonic exercise). Sounds ridiculously simple, but can such easy motions really help patellar tendinitis? Surprisingly, *yes…*

- 29 volleyball and basketball players with patellar tendinitis, currently either playing or training, were randomly assigned to one of two groups (Van Ark 2016)

- the first group performed *isometric* contractions on a leg extension machine

- the second group did *isotonic* contractions on a leg extension machine

- both groups continued with their matches and training sessions

- after 4-weeks, pain significantly improved in both groups, with no significant differences between the two groups

Perhaps the best thing about this study, is that it took athletes that had patellar tendinitis and got them better – *despite the fact that they continued to play, train, and compete* – which is pretty darn impressive considering the stress that the patellar tendon is under when it comes to jumping sports such as basketball and volleyball!

The next few pages will show you how to do the **isometric** and **isotonic** exercises on a leg extension machine…

The Leg Extension Machine and Finding Your One Repetition Maximum (1 RM)

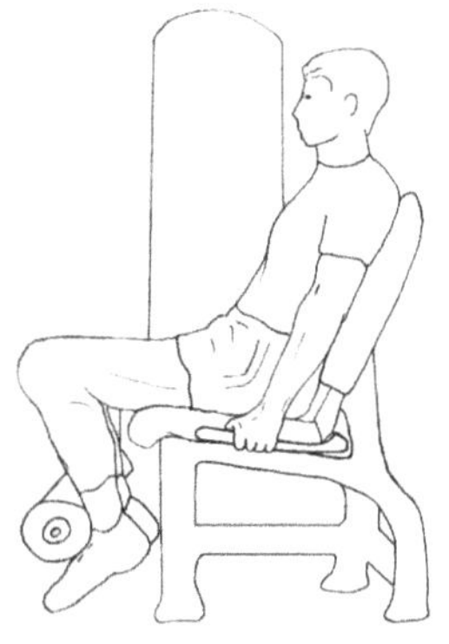

- the ISOMETRIC leg extension exercise is done on a leg extension machine and has you use a weight that is a percentage of your 1 RM – so you will first need to find your 1 RM

- position yourself in the leg extension machine as the picture shows. If you are unfamiliar with this machine, it is suggested that you first consult with knowledgeable staff at your gym to get familiar

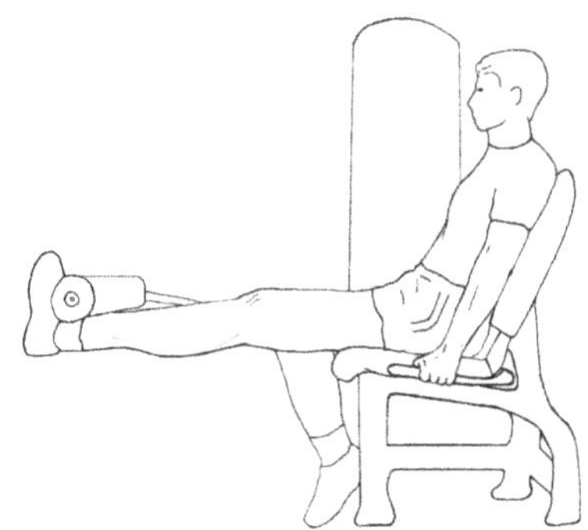

- set the machine on a light weight and kick your leg out straight like the picture shows, and then back down. Do this about 10 times in order to warm up.

- rest for a minute or two, and then take a guess at the amount of weight you think you can lift once, and only once, in good form. Good form is kicking your leg out straight in about 2-3 seconds, and then lowering it back down in about 2-3 seconds.

- if you could only lift that weight once, that's your 1 RM. If not, rest several minutes, and then try again after either adding or subtracting weight – depending if you did more than one rep – or couldn't do one at all.

- repeat this process as needed until you find your 1 RM – the weight you can lift once, and only once, in good form

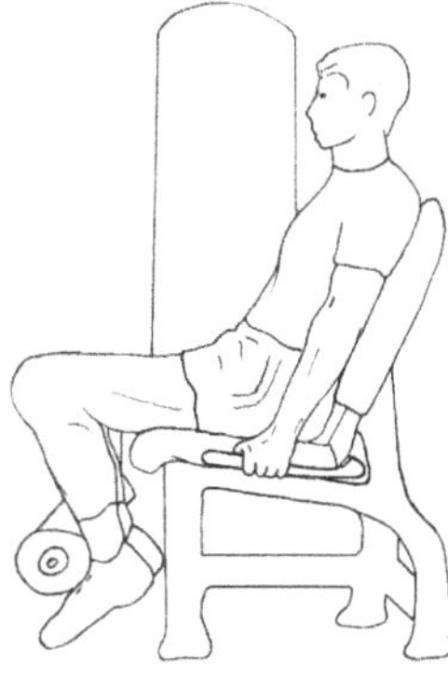

- when you determine how many pounds is your 1 RM, you will need to find out how many pounds is 80% of that – because that's the weight you'll be using to do the isometric leg extension exercise. To do this, multiply your 1 RM by .8

- for example, if your 1 RM was 100 pounds, 100 x .8 = 80. Therefore, you will be using 80 pounds to do the isometric leg extension exercise on the next page.

Isometric Leg Extension Exercise

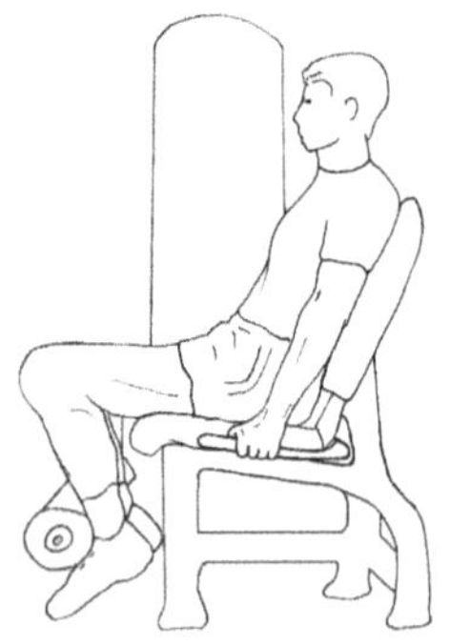

- first, set the weight on the machine to the weight you determined to be 80% of your 1 RM. Using the example from the previous page, you would set the machine on 80 pounds.
- position yourself on the leg extension machine as the picture shows.

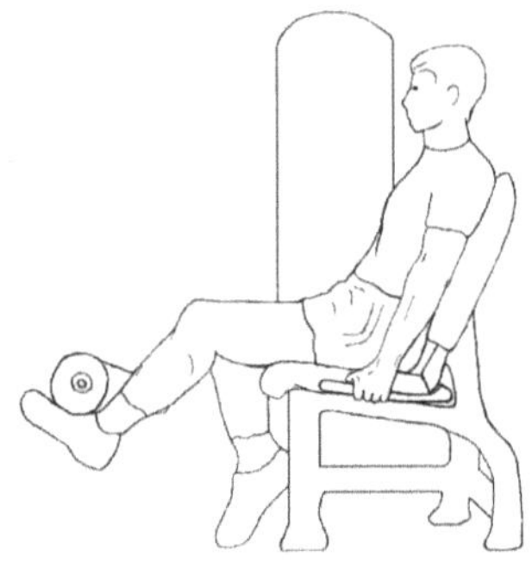

- next, kick your leg out to around a 45-degree angle as the picture shows
- hold it there for 45 seconds

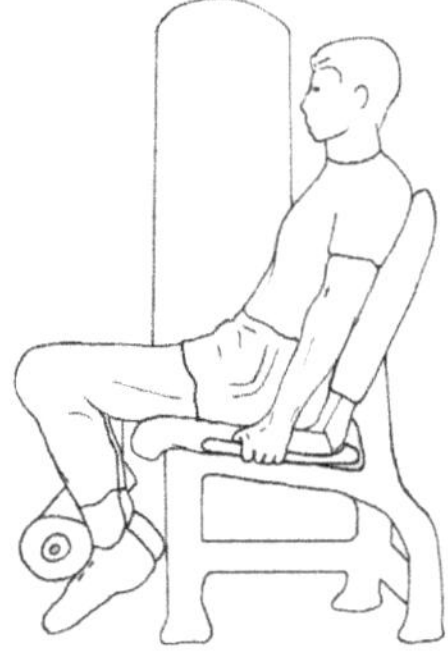

- return to the starting position as the picture shows, and rest for about 1 minute
- repeat this 4 more times. In total, you will be holding your leg out 5 times for 45 seconds (5 x 45s) each session.
- do the same with your other leg if you have patellar tendinitis in it too
- do this session four times a week on days that are convenient for you
- add a pound or two a week if possible
- if pain is experienced, or you are unable to complete a repetition in good form, lower the weight for the following repetitions so you can complete the entire session. Continue for 4 weeks.

The Leg Extension Machine and Finding Your Eight Repetition Maximum (8 RM)

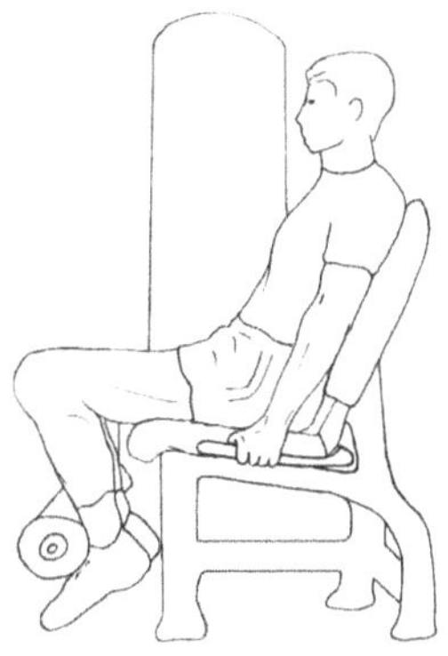

- the ISOTONIC leg extension exercise is done on a leg extension machine and has you use a weight that is a percentage of your 8 RM – so you will first need to find your 8 RM

- position yourself in the leg extension machine as the picture shows. If you are unfamiliar with this machine, it is suggested that you first consult with knowledgeable staff at your gym to get familiar

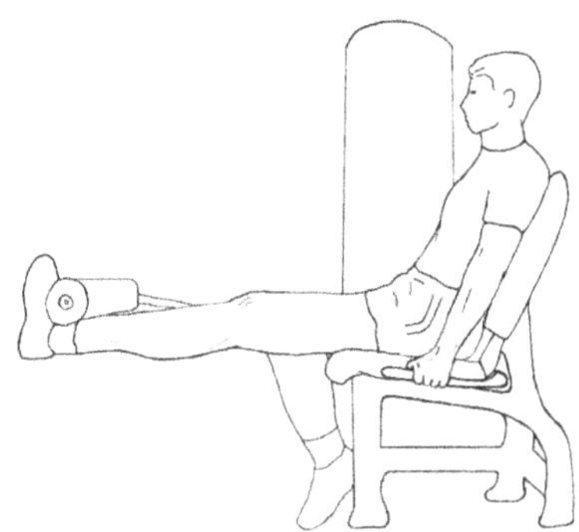

- set the machine on a light weight and kick your leg out straight like the picture shows, and then back down. Do this about 10 times in order to warm up.

- rest for a minute or two, and then take a guess at the amount of weight you think you can lift 8 times, and only 8 times, in good form. Good form is kicking your leg out straight in about 2–3 seconds, and then lowering it back down in about 2–3 seconds.

- if you could only lift that weight 8 times, that's your 8 RM. If not, rest several minutes, and then try again after either adding or subtracting weight – depending if you did more or less than 8 times.

- repeat this process as needed until you find your 8 RM – the weight you can lift 8 times, and only 8 times, in good form

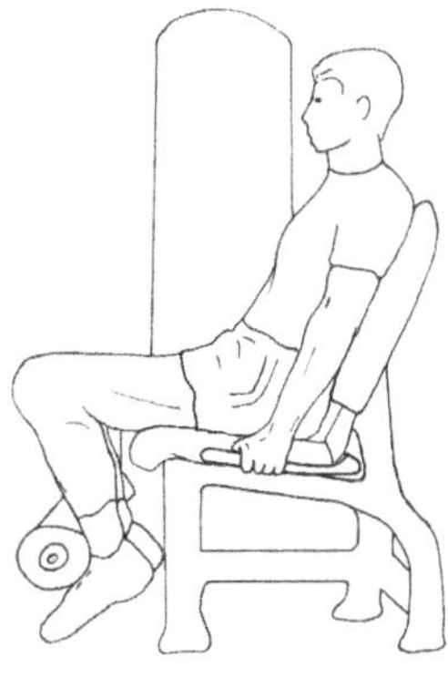

- when you determine how many pounds is your 8 RM, you will need to find out how many pounds is 80% of that – because that's the weight you'll be using to do the isotonic leg extension exercise. To do this, multiply your 8 RM by .8

- for example, if your 8 RM was 50 pounds, 50 x .8 = 40. Therefore, you will be using 40 pounds to do the isotonic leg extension exercise on the next page.

Isotonic Leg Extension Exercise

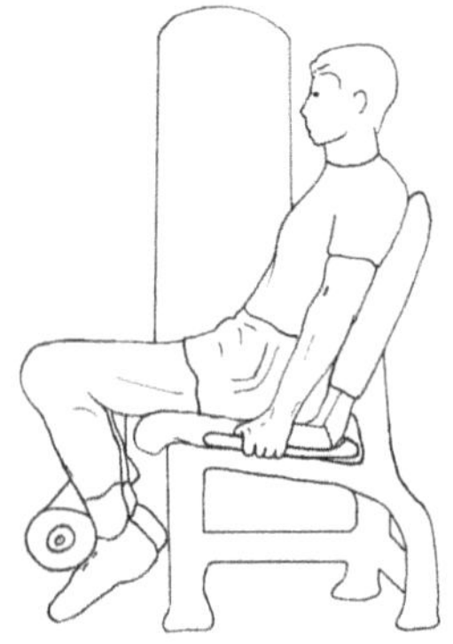

- first, set the weight on the machine to the weight you determined to be 80% of your 8 RM. Using the example from the previous page, you would set the machine on 40 pounds.
- position yourself on the leg extension machine as the picture shows.

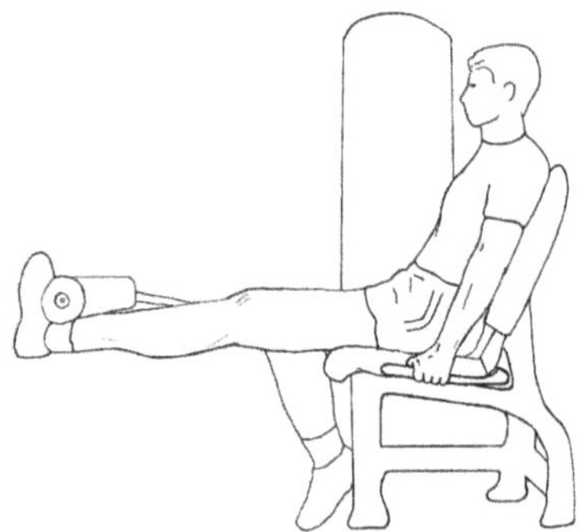

- next, kick your leg out until your knee is straight, then lower it back down
- it should take you about 3 seconds to kick your leg out, and about 4 seconds to lower it back down
- repeat this 7 more times. In total, you will be kicking your leg out 8 times in a row each set.
- after doing a set of 8 reps, rest for about a minute - and then repeat this 3 more times. Therefore, you will be doing 4 sets of 8 repetitions (4 x 8 reps), with a minute of rest in between sets.

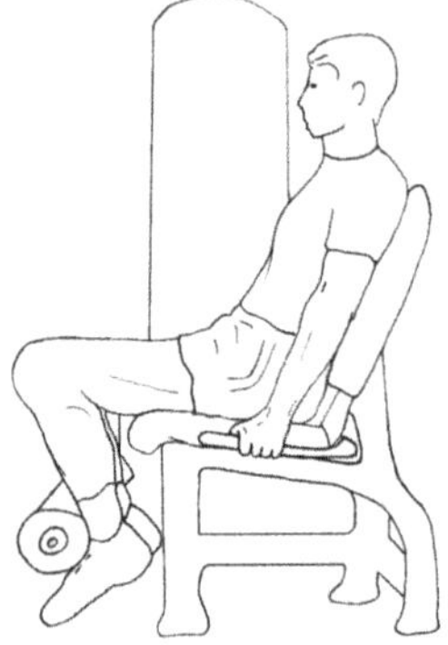

- do the same with your other leg if you have patellar tendinitis in it too
- do this session (4 x 8 reps) four times a week on days that are convenient for you
- add a pound or two a week if possible
- if pain is experienced, or you are unable to complete repetitions in good form, lower the weight for the following repetitions so you can complete the entire session. Continue for 4 weeks.

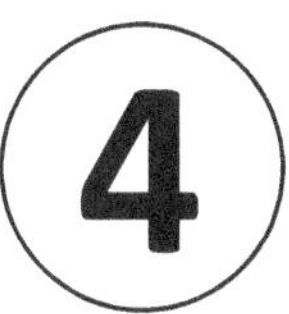

RE-CAP

As mentioned earlier, the highest form of proof in medicine that a treatment is actually effective, or "works", is the randomized controlled trial. And, as you have read in the previous pages, we have plenty of them showing us that certain knee exercises can, in fact, help tremendously with patellar tendonitis. Here's a quick re-cap of the evidence-based strengthening exercise options we've just covered - along with a few comments…

Eccentric Decline Squats

This is probably one of the easiest to try, as it requires very little equipment. You will need a slant board - they are easy to find online, and are usually made of either plastic or wood. Most are adjustable, meaning that you can set them at different angles.

Recall that most studies using the eccentric decline squat to fix patellar tendinitis have used the 25-degree slant board. Now does that mean you have to run out and get *precisely* a 25-degree slant board? Not really. It would be my first choice, but as the study on page 30 shows us, any slant board angle between 15-degrees and 30-degrees will work quite sufficiently to increase patellar tendon force – and thus can be used to do this exercise.

As far as equipment, the only other thing you would need is a backpack. That way, as you progress, and can do 3 sets of 15 reps with minimal to no pain, you simply load up a backpack with 10 pounds when doing the squats - in order to keep a sufficient load on the patellar tendon.

With the simplicity of the exercise and equipment, the eccentric decline squat is my go-to home exercise for patellar tendinitis.

Heavy Slow Resistance Exercises

This is the most involved of the four. First of all, it does require a motivated individual. That's because you have to do three different exercises – and multiple sets of each. Additionally, you also have to go to a gym to do them – and you have to find a gym that has certain machines, such as the hack squat machine. While far from impossible to find, not all gyms have one.

Perhaps most daunting of all, is finding your specific repetition maximum for a given week. It does take trial and error, but one thing to point out. Once you find your 15RM, it will be much easier to find your 12RM. Likewise, once you know your 12RM, you'll be able to take a pretty accurate guess at to what your 10RM might be – and so there's less trial and error involved as the program progresses. Like I said, it does sound tedious, but once you figure out a few of your RM's, the rest get easier to find.

So those are possible disadvantages for some. The big advantage, however, is that heavy slow resistance training has shown to be well worth the effort. Long-term follow-up show us that people with patellar tendinitis are much more satisfied with the results when using this specific method compared to eccentric decline squats. Furthermore, when biopsies of patellar tendons are compared, heavy slow resistance exercise produces the most normal looking tendons of all.

The bottom line is that if you like to work out, and have access to a gym – this would be a great option.

Isometric Leg Extensions

The isometric leg extension exercise is by far the most *time-efficient* exercise you can do to get rid of your patellar tendinitis. The actual time you spend exercising is 45 seconds x 5 reps, which is around 4 minutes. Now add a minute of rest in between each set, and you can see how one can easily complete a session in well under 10 minutes a day! Even better, you just do four sessions a week *on days that are convenient* – so no strict workout schedules here.

Disadvantages are few, for instance you'll have to make it to a gym and use a leg extension machine. But, these aren't hard to find at all - and I can't think of the last time I worked out in a gym that didn't have one. Other than that, the only other issue is that you can't just hop on the leg extension machine and begin - that is you'll have to find your 1RM first. But once you find it, you're set for the rest of the program – just add a pound or two each week as tolerated.

So if you're not into exercise, or have a hectic schedule, the isometric leg extension exercise is a good choice.

Isotonic Leg Extensions

The isotonic leg extension exercise has the same disadvantages as the *isometric* exercise – for instance you can't do it at home, and you have to find your 8RM first before beginning. Yet another disadvantage is that it requires a bit more time in the gym. Instead of doing five 45-second holds, you're going to be doing 4 sets of 8 reps - however, it's still a pretty small investment of your time to fix your patellar tendon with just *one exercise*.

Consider this option if you can get to a gym and prefer full range of motion exercise over isometric holds.

Evidence-Based Exercises for Patellar Tendinitis

❯ Eccentric Decline Squats
❯ Heavy Slow Resistance Exercises
❯ Isometric Leg Extension Exercise
❯ Isotonic Leg Extension Exercise

---

⑤

SUPPORTING REFERENCES

It's true! All the information in this book is based on *randomized controlled trials* and scientific studies that have been published in peer-reviewed journals. Since I know there are readers out there like myself that like to actually check out the information for themselves, I've included the references for *every* study I have cited in this book (in alphabetical order). *Never* trust a self-help book that doesn't have sound research to support its advice…

Alfredson H, et al. In vivo microdialysis and immunohistochemical analyses of tendon tissue demonstrated high amounts of free glutamate and glutamate NMDAR1 receptors, but no signs of inflammation, in jumper's knee. *Journal of Orthopaedic Research* 2001;19:881-886.

Alfredson H, et al. Superior results with eccentric compared to concentric quadriceps training in patients with jumper's knee: a prospective randomised study. *Br J Sports Med* 2005;39:847-850.

Bahr R, et al. Surgical treatment compared with eccentric training for patellar tendinopathy (jumper's knee). A randomized, controlled trial. *Journal of Bone and Joint Surgery* 2006;88-A:1689-1698.

Fu S, et al. Increased expression of transforming growth factor-B1 in patellar tendinosis. *Clinical Orthopaedics and Related Research* 2002;400:174-183.

Khan K, et al. Patellar tendinosis (jumper's knee): findings at histopathologic examination, US and MR imaging. *Radiology* 1996;200:821-827.

Kongsgaard M, et al. Corticosteroid injections, eccentric decline squat training, and heavy slow resistance training in patellar tendinopathy. *Scandinavian Journal of Medicine and Science in Sports* 2009;19:790-802.

Popp J, et al. Recalcitrant patellar tendinitis. Magnetic resonance imaging, histologic evaluation, and surgical treatment. *American Journal of Sports Medicine* 1997;25:218-222.

Van Ark M, et al. Do isometric and isotonic exercise programs reduce pain in athletes with patellar tendinopathy in-season? A randomised clinical trial. *Journal of Science and Medicine in Sport* 2016;19:702-706.

Yu J, et al. Correlation of MR imaging and pathologic findings in athletes undergoing surgery for chronic patellar tendinitis. *AJR* 1995:165:115-118.

Zwerver J, et al. Biomechanical analysis of the single-leg decline squat. *Br J Sports Med* 2007;41:264-268.